DIARY OF A NURSING SISTER

ANON

AMBERLEY

This edition first published 2014

Amberley Publishing
The Hill, Stroud
Gloucestershire, GL5 4EP

www.amberley-books.com

British Library Cataloguing in Publication Data.
A catalogue record for this book is available from the British Library.

ISBN 978 1 4456 4197 3 (print)
ISBN 978 1 4456 4205 5 (ebook)

Typeset in 10pt on 12pt Sabon.
Typesetting and Origination by Amberley Publishing.
Printed in the UK.

DIARY
OF A
NURSING
SISTER

CONTENTS

Waiting for Orders

August 18, 1914, to September 14, 1914

The voyage out—Havre—Leaving Havre—R.M.S.P.
Asturias—St Nazaire—Orders at last.

S.S. *City of Benares* (troopship)

Tuesday, 8 p.m., August 18th.
Orders just gone round that there are to be no lights after dark,
so I am hasting to write this.

We had a great send-off in Sackville Street in our motor-bus,
and went on board about 2 p.m. From then till 7 we watched
the embarkation going on, on our own ship and another. We
have a lot of R.E. and R.F.A. and A.S.C., and a great many
horses and pontoons and ambulance waggons: the horses were
very difficult to embark, poor dears. It was an exciting scene
all the time. I don't remember anything quite so thrilling as
our start off from Ireland. All the 600 khaki men on board,
and every one on every other ship, and all the crowds on the
quay, and in boats and on lighthouses, waved and yelled. Then
we and the officers and the men, severally, had the King's
proclamation read out to us about doing our duty for our
country, and God blessing us, and how the King is following
our every movement.

We are now going to snatch up a very scratch supper and
turn in, only rugs and blankets.

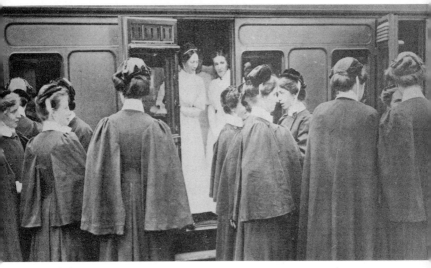

English nurses entraining.

Wednesday, August 19th.
We are having a lovely calm and sunny voyage – slowed down
in the night for a fog. I had a berth by an open port-hole, and
though rather cold with one blanket and a rug (dressing-gown
in my trunk), enjoyed it very much – cold sea bath in the
morning. We live on oatmeal biscuits and potted meat, with
chocolate and tea and soup squares, some bread and butter
sometimes, and cocoa at bed-time.

There is a routine by bugle-call on troopships, with a guard,
police, and fatigues. The Tommies sleep on bales of forage in
the after well-deck and all over the place. We have one end of
the 1st class cabin forrard, and the officers have the 2nd class
aft for sleeping and meals, but there is a sociable blend on deck
all day. Two medical officers here were both in South Africa at
No. 7 when I was (Captains in those days), and we have had
great cracks on old times and all the people we knew. One is
commanding a Field Ambulance and goes with the fighting
line. There are 200 men for Field Ambulances on board. They
don't carry Sisters, worse luck, only Padres.

We had an impromptu service on deck this afternoon; I played the hymns,—never been on a voyage yet without being let in for that. It was run by the three C. of E. Padres and the Wesleyan hand in hand: the latter has been in the Nile Expedition of '98 and all through South Africa. We had Mission Hymns roared by the Tommies, and then a C. of E. Padre gave a short address – quite good. The Wesleyan did an extempore prayer, rather well, and a very nice huge C. of E. man gave the Blessing. Now they are having a Tommies' concert – a talented boy at the piano.

At midday we passed a French cruiser, going the opposite way. They waved and yelled, and we waved and yelled. We are out of sight of English or French coast now. I believe we are to be in early to-morrow morning, and will have a long train journey probably, but nobody knows anything for certain except where we land – Havre.

It seems so long since we heard anything about the war, but it is only since yesterday morning. (The concert is rather distracting, and the wind is getting up – one of the Tommies has an angelic black puppy on his lap, with a red cross on its collar, and there is a black cat about.)

Thursday, August 20th, 5 p.m., Havre.
We got in about 9 o'clock this morning. Havre is a very picturesque town, with very high houses, and a great many docks and quays, and an enormous amount of shipping. The wharves were as usual lined with waving yelling crowds, and a great exchange of Vive l'Angleterre from them, and Vive la France from us went on, and a lusty roar of the Marseillaise from us. During the morning the horses and pontoons and waggons were disembarked, and the R.E. and Field Ambulances went off to enormous sheds on the wharf. We went off in a taxi in batches of five to the Convent de St Jeanne d'Arc, an enormous empty school, totally devoid of any furniture except crucifixes! Luckily the school washhouse has quite good basins and taps, and we are all camping out, three in a room, to sleep on the floor, as our camp kit isn't available. No one knows if we shall be here one night, or a week, or for ever! It is a glorious

place, with huge high rooms, and huge open casements, and broad staircases and halls, windows looking over the town to the sea. We are high up on a hill. There's no food here, so we sit on the floor and make our own breakfast and tea, and go to a very swanky hotel for lunch and dinner. We are billeted here for quarters, and at the hotel for meals.

A room full of mattresses has just been discovered to our joy, and we have all hauled one up to our rooms, so we shall be in luxury.

Just got a French paper and seen the Pope is dead, and a very enthusiastic account of the British troops at Dunkerque, their marvellous organisation, their cheerfulness, and their behaviour.

Just seen on the Official War News placarded in the town that the Germans have crossed the Meuse between Liège and Namur, and the Belgians are retiring on to Antwerp. The Allies must buck up.

The whole town is flying flags since the troops began to come in; all the biggest shops and buildings fly all four of the Allies.

Friday, August 21st.
Intercession Day at home. There is a beautiful chapel in the Convent.

There is almost as much censoring about the movement of the French troops in the French papers as there is about ours in the English, and not a great deal about the movements of the Germans.

There are 43 Sisters belonging to No.— General Hospital on the floor below us camping out in the same way – 86 altogether in the building, one wing of which is the Sick Officers' Hospital of No.— G.H.

The No.— people are moving up the line to-night. It will take a few days to get No.— together, and then we shall move on at night. The Colonel knows where to, but he has not told Matron; she thinks it will be farther up than Amiens or Rheims, where two more have already gone, but it is all guess-work. I expect No.— from C—— is in Belgium. (It was at Amiens and had to leave in a hurry.)

The whole system of Field Medical Service has altered since South Africa. The wounded are picked up on the field by the *regimental stretcher-bearers*, who are generally the band, trained in First Aid and Stretcher Drill. They take them to the Bearer Section of the *Field Ambulance* (which used to be called Field Hospital), who take them to the Tent Section of the same Field Ambulance, who have been getting the *Dressing Station* ready with sterilisers, &c., while the Bearer Section are fetching them from the regimental stretcher-bearers. They are all drilled to get this ready in twenty minutes in tents, but it takes longer in farmhouses. The Field Ambulance then takes them in ambulance waggons (with lying down and sitting accommodation) to the *Clearing Hospital*, with beds, and returns empty to the Dressing Station. From the Clearing Hospital they go on to the *Stationary Hospital* – 200 beds – which is on a railway, and finally in hospital trains to the *General Hospital*, their last stopping-place before they get shipped off to *Netley* and all the English hospitals. The General Hospitals are the only ones at present to carry Sisters; 500 beds is the minimum, and they are capable of expanding indefinitely.

There is a large staff of harassed-looking landing officers here, with a.m.L.O. on a white armband for the medical people; a great many troopships are coming from Southampton; you hear them booing their signals in the harbour all night and day.

I've had my first letter from England, from a patient at ——. The Field Service post-card is quite good as a means of communication, but frightfully tantalising from our point of view.

We had a very good night on our mattresses, but it was rather cold towards morning with only one rug.

They have a Carter-Paterson motor-van for the Military mail-cart at the M.P.O., and two Tommies sit by a packing-case with a slit in the lid for the letter-box.

Saturday, August 22nd.
The worst has happened. No.— is to stop at Havre; in camp three miles out. So No.— and No.— are both staying here.

Meanwhile to-day Nos.—, —, and— have all arrived; 130 more Sisters besides the 86 already here are packed into this Convent, camping out in dining-halls and schoolrooms and passages. The big Chapel below and the wee Chapel on this floor seem to be the only unoccupied places now.

Havre is a big base for the France part of our Expeditionary Force. Troopships are arriving every day, and every fighting man is being hurried up to the Front, and they cannot block the lines and trains with all these big hospitals yet.

The news from the Front looks bad to-day – Namur under heavy fire, and the Germans pressing on Antwerp, and the French chased out of Lorraine.

Everybody is hoping it doesn't mean staying here permanently, but you never know your luck. It all depends what happens farther up, and of course one might have the luck to be added to a hospital farther up to fill up casualties among Sisters or if more were wanted.

The base hospitals, of course, are always filling up from up country with men who may be able to return to duty, and acute or hopeless cases who have to be got well enough for a hospital ship for home.

There is to be a Requiem Mass to-morrow at Notre Dame for those who have been killed in the war, and the whole nave and choir is reserved for officials and Red Cross people. It is a most beautiful church, now hung all over with the four flags of the Allies. An old woman in the church this morning asked us if we were going to the Blessés, and clasped our hands and blessed us and wept. She must have had some sons in the army.

We are simply longing to get to work, whether here or anywhere else; it is 100 per cent better in this interesting old town doing for ourselves in the Convent than waiting in the stuffy hotel at Dublin. There is any amount to see – miles of our Transport going through the town with burly old shaggy English farm-horses, taken straight from the harvest, pulling the carts; French Artillery Reservists being taught to work the guns; French soldiers passing through; and our R.E.

Motor-cyclists scudding about. And one can practise talking, understanding, and reading French. It is surprising how few of the 216 Sisters here seem to know a word of French. I am looked upon as an expert, and you know what my French is like! A sick officer sitting out in the court below has got a small French boy by him who is teaching him French with a map, a 'Matin,' and a dictionary. A great deal of nodding and shaking of heads is going on.

Sunday, August 23rd.

The same dazzling blue sky, boiling sun, and sharp shadows that one seldom sees in England for long together; we've had it for days.

We've had yesterday's London papers to read to-day; they quote in a rather literal translation from their Paris Correspondent word for word what we read in the Paris papers yesterday. I wonder what the English hospital people in Brussels are doing in the German occupation – pretty hard times for them, I expect. Two that I know are there doing civilian work, and Lord Rothschild has got a lot of English nurses there.

This morning I went to the great Requiem Mass at Notre Dame. It was packed to bursting with people standing, but we were immediately shown to good places. The Abbé preached a very fine war sermon, quite easy to understand. There was a great deal of weeping on all sides. When the service was finished the big organ suddenly struck up 'God Save the King'; it gave one such a thrill. And then a long procession of officers filed out, our generals with three rows of ribbons leading, and the French following.

This is said to be our biggest base, and that we shall get some very good work. Of course, once we get the wounded in it doesn't make any difference where you are.

Monday, August 24th.

The news looks bad to-day; people say it is très sérieux, ce moment-ci; but there is a cheering article in Saturday's Times about it all. The news is posted up at the Préfeture (dense crowd always) several times a day, and we get many editions of the papers as we go through the day.

Tuesday, August 25th.
We bide here. No.— G.H., which is also here, has been chopped in half, and divided between us and No.— General, the permanent Base Hospital already established here. So we shall be two base hospitals, each with 750 beds.

The place is full of rumours of all sorts of horrors – that the Germans have landed in Scotland, that they are driving the Allies back on all sides, and that the casualties are in thousands. So far there are 200 sick, minor cases, at No.—, but no wounded except two Germans. We have no beds open yet; the hospital is still being got on with; our site is said to be on a swamp between a Remount Camp and a Veterinary Camp, so we shall do well in horse-flies.

It is a fortnight to-morrow since we mobilised, and we have had no work yet except our own fatigue duty in the Convent; it was our turn this morning, and I scrubbed the lavatories out with creosol.

I've had an interesting day to-day, motoring round with the C.O. of No.— and the No.— Matron. We visited each of their three palatial buildings in turn, huge wards of 60 beds each, in ball-rooms, and a central camp of 500 on a hill outside. They have their work cut out having it so divided up, but they are running it magnificently.

Wednesday, August 26th.
Very ominous leading articles in the French papers to-day bidding everyone to remember that there is no need to give up hope of complete success in the end! There is a great deal about the French and English heavy losses, but where are the wounded being sent? It is absolutely maddening sitting here still with no work yet, when there must be so much to be done; but I suppose it will come to us in time, as it is easier to move the men to the hospitals than the hospitals to the men, or they wouldn't have put 1500 beds here.

The street children here have a charming way of running up to every strolling Tommy, Officer, or Sister, seizing their hand, and saying, 'Goodnight,' and saluting; one reached up to pat my shoulder.

No.— G.H., which left here yesterday for Abbeville, between Rouen and the mouth of the Somme, came back again to-day. They were met by a telegram at Rouen at midnight, telling them to return to Havre, as it was not safe to go on. They are of course frightfully sick.

French wounded have been coming in all day. And we are not yet in camp. Our site is said to be a fearful swamp, so to-day, which has been soaking wet, will be a good test for it.

It is so wet to-night that we are going to have cocoa and bread-and-butter on the floor, instead of trailing down to the hotel for dinner. Miss ——, who is the third in our room, regales us with really thrilling stories of her adventures in S.A. She was mentioned in despatches, and reported dead.

Thursday, August 27th.

Bright sun to-day, so I hope the Army is drying itself. All sorts of rumours as usual – that our wounded are still on the field, being shot by the Germans, that 700 are coming to Havre to-day, that 700 have been taken in at Rouen, where we have three G.H.'s – that last is the truest story. We went this afternoon to see over the Hospital Ship here, waiting for wounded to take back to Netley. It is beautifully fitted, and even has hot-water bottles ready in the beds, but no wounded. It is much smaller than the H.S. *Dunera* I came home in from South Africa. Still no sign of No.— being ready, which is not surprising, as the hay had to be cut and the place drained more or less. The French and English officers here all sit at different tables, and don't hobnob much. Six officers of the Royal Flying Corps are here, double-breasted tunics and two spread-eagle wings on left breast. Troops are still arriving at the docks, which are the biggest I have ever seen. The men on the trams give us back our sous, as we are 'Militaires.'

Friday, August 28th.

Hot and brilliant. Eleven fugitive Sisters of No.— have come back to-day from Amiens, and the others are either hung up somewhere or on the way. The story is that Uhlans were arriving in the town, and that it wasn't safe for women; I don't know if the hospital were receiving wounded or not. Yes, they were. Another rumour to-day says that No.— Field Ambulance has been wiped out by a bomb from an aeroplane. Another rumour says that one regiment has five men left, and another one man – but most of these stories turn out myths in time.

Wounded are being taken in at No.—, and are being shipped home from there the same day.

This morning Matron took two of us out to our Hospital camp, three miles along the Harfleur road. The tram threaded its way through thousands of our troops, who arrived this morning, and through a regiment of French Sappers. There were Seaforths (with khaki petticoats over the kilt), R. Irish Rifles, R.B. Gloucesters, Connaughts, and some D.G.'s and Lancers. They were all heavily loaded up with kit and rifles (sometimes a proud little French boy would carry these for them), marching well, but perspiring in rivers. It was a good sight, and the contrast between the khaki and the red trousers and caps and blue coats of the French was very striking. We went nearly to Harfleur (where Henry V. landed before Agincourt), and then walked back towards No.— Camp, along a beautiful straight avenue with poplars meeting over the top. About 20 motors full of Belgian officers passed us.

The camp is getting on well. All the Hospital tents are pitched, and all the quarters except the Sisters and the big store tents for the Administration block are ready. The operating theatre tent is to have a concrete floor and is not ready.

The ground is the worst part. It is a very boggy hay-field, and in wet weather like Wednesday and Tuesday they say it is a swamp. We are all to have our skirts and aprons very short and to be well provided with gum-boots. We shall be two in a bell-tent, or dozens in a big store tent, uncertain yet which, and we are to have a bath tent. I am to be surgical.

While waiting for the tram on the way back, on a hot, white road, we made friends with a French soldier, who stopped a little motor-lorry, already crammed with men and some sort of casks, and made them take us on. I sat on the floor, with my feet on the step, and we whizzed back into Havre in great style. There is no speed limit, and it was a lovely joy-ride!

We are seeing the Times a few days late and fairly regularly. Have not seen any list of the Charleroi casualties yet. It all seems to be coming much nearer now. The line is very much taken up with ammunition trains.

To show that there is a good deal going on, though we've as yet had no work, I'm only half through my 7d. book, and we left home a fortnight and two days ago. If you do have a chance to read anything but newspapers, you can't keep your mind on it.

We are getting quite used to a life shorn of most of its trappings, except for the two hotel meals a day.

My mattress, on the floor along the very low large window, with two rugs and cushions, and a holdall for a bolster, is as comfortable as any bed, and you don't miss sheets after a day or two. There is one bathroom for 120 or more people, but I get a cold bath every morning early. S—— gets our early morning tea, and M. sweeps our room, and I wash up and roll up the beds. We are still away from our boxes, and have a change of some clothes and not others. I have to wash my vest overnight when I want a clean one and put it on in the morning. We have slung a clothes-line across our room. The view is absolutely glorious.

Saturday, August 29th.
A grilling day. It is very difficult, this waiting. No.— had 450 wounded in yesterday, and they were whisked off on the hospital ship in the evening. It doesn't look as if there would be anything for us to do for weeks.

Sunday, August 30th.
Orders to-day for the whole Base at Havre to pack itself up

and embark at a moment's notice. So No.—, No.—, No.—, and No.— G.H., who are all here, and a Royal Flying Corps unit, the Post Office, and the Staff, and every blessed British unit, are all packing up for dear life. We may be going home, and we may be going to Brittany, to Cherbourg, or to Brest, or to Berlin.

Monday, August 31st.
We all got up at 5.30 to be ready, but I daresay we shan't move to-day. Yesterday we had two starved, exhausted, fugitive (from Amiens) No.— Sisters in to tea on our floor, and heard their stories. The last seventeen of them fled with the wounded. A train of cattle-trucks came in at Rouen with all the wounded as they were picked up without a spot of dressing on any of their wounds, which were septic and full of straw and dirt. The matron, M.O., and some of them got hold of some dressings and went round doing what they could in the time, and others fed them. Then the No.— got their Amiens wounded into cattle-trucks on mattresses, with Convent pillows, and had a twenty hours' journey with them in frightful smells and dirt. Our visitor had five badly-wounded officers, one shot through the lungs and hip, and all full of bullets and spunk. They were magnificent, and asked riddles and whistled, and the men were the same. They'd been travelling already for two days. An orderly fell out of the train and was badly injured, and died next morning.

It is very interesting to read on Monday *The Times'* Military Correspondent's forecast of Friday. He seems to know so exactly the different lines of defence of the Allies, and exactly where the Germans will try and break through. But he has never found out that Havre has been a base for over a fortnight. He speaks of Havre or Cherbourg as a possible base to fall back upon, if fortified against long-distance artillery firing, which we are not. And now we are abandoning Havre!

Tuesday, September 1st.
No orders yet, so we are still waiting, packed up.

Went with one of the regulars to-day to see the big hospital ship *Asturias* with 3000 beds, and also to see Sister — at the No.— Maritime Hospital. They've been very busy there dressing the wounded for the ship. Colonel — brought us back in his motor, and met the Consul-General on the way, who told us K. came through today off a cruiser, and was taken on to Paris in a motor. Smiles of relief from everyone. One of the Sisters had heard from her mother in Scotland that she had five Russian officers billeted! They are said to be on their way through from Archangel.

Troopships full of French and English troops are leaving Havre every day, for Belgium.

Wouldn't you like to be under the table when K. and J. and F. are poring over their maps to-night?

Wednesday, September 2nd.

We are leaving to-morrow, on a hospital ship, possibly for Nantes. K. has given orders for everyone to be cleared out of Havre by to-morrow.

We found some men invalided from the Front lying outside the station last night waiting for an ambulance, mostly reservists called up; they'd had a hot time, but were full of grit.

The men from Mons told us 'it wasn't fighting – it was murder'. They said the burning hot sun was one of the worst parts. They said 'the officers was grand'; many regiments seem to have hardly any officers left. They all say that the S. A. War was a picnic compared to this German artillery onslaught and their packed masses continually filling up.

There is a darling little chapel on this floor, beautifully kept, just as the nuns left it, where one can say one's prayers. And there is also a lovely church, where they have Mass at 8 every morning.

You can imagine how hard it has been to keep off grumbling at not getting any work all this time; it is one of the worst of fortunes of war. It seems as if most of the 'dangerously' and many of the 'seriously' wounded must have died pretty soon, or have not been picked up. The cases that do come down are most of them slight. Some of the worst must be in hospital at Rouen.

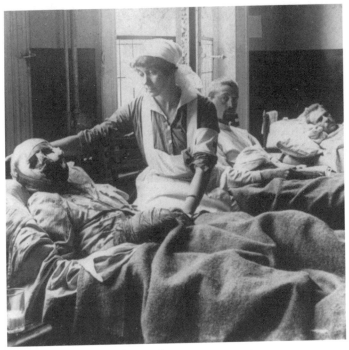

The badly-wounded in hospital.

Friday, September 4th. R.M.S.P. Asturias, *Havre.*
At last we are uprooted from that convent up the hot hill
and are on an enormous hospital ship, who in times of peace
goes to New York and Brazil and the Argentine. There are 240
Sisters on her, one or two M.O.'s, and all the No.— equipment.
She is like a great white town; you can walk for miles on her
decks; she is the biggest I have ever been on; we are in the
cabins, and the wards and operating-theatres are all equipped
for patients, but at the moment she is being used as a transport
for us. We are supposed to be going to St Nazaire, the port
for Nantes. They can't possibly be going to dump No.—,
No.—, No.—, No.—, and No.— all down at the new base, so
I suppose one or two of the hospitals will be sent up the new
lines of communication.

Poor Havre is very desolate. All the flags came down when the British left, and the people looked very sad. Paris refugees are crowding in, and sleeping on the floors of the hotels, and camping out in their motor cars, and many crossing to England. There is a Proclamation up all over the town telling the people to pull themselves together whatever happens, and to forget everything that is not La Patrie. Also another about the military necessity for the Government to leave Paris, and that they mustn't be afraid of anything that may happen, because we shall win in the end, &c., &c.

We don't start till to-morrow, I believe; meanwhile, cleanliness and privacy and sheets, and cool, quick meals and sea breeze, are cheering after the grime and the pigging and the squash and the awful heat of the last fortnight. I have picked up a bad cold from the foul dust-heaps and drainless condition of the smelly Havre streets, but it will soon disappear now.

I wish I could tell you the extraordinary beauty of yesterday evening from the ship. There was a flaming sunset below a pale-green sky, and then the thousand lights of the ships and the town came out reflected in the water, and then a brilliant moon. A big American cruiser was alongside of us.

We shall get no more letters till we land. I have a 'State-room' all to myself on the top deck; the waiters and stewards are English, very polite to us, and the crew are mostly West African negroes, who talk good English. The ship is very becoming to the white, grey, and red of our uniforms, or else our uniforms are becoming to the ship, and her many decks; but why, oh why, are we not all in hospital somewhere?

Saturday, September 5th.
Had a perfect voyage – getting in to Nantes to-night – after that no one knows. Shouldn't be surprised if we are sent home.

La Baule, near Nantes.

Monday, September 7th.

The latest wave of this erratic sea has tossed us up on to two little French seaside places north of St Nazaire, the port of Nantes. There are over 500 Sisters at the two places in hotels. No.— and No.— and part of — are at La Baule in one enormous new hotel, which has been taken over for the French wounded on the bottom floor; the rest was empty till we came. We are in palatial rooms with balconies overlooking the sea, and have large bathrooms opening out of our rooms; it is rather like the Riffel in the middle of a forest of pines, and the sea immediately in front. The expense of it all must be colossal! Every one is too sick at the state of affairs to enjoy it at all; some bathe, and you can sit about in the pines or on the sands. We have had no letters since we left Havre last Thursday, and no news of the war. We took till Sunday morning to reach St Nazaire, and at midday were stuffed into a little dirty train for this place. I'm thankful we didn't have to get out at Pornichet, the station before this, where are Nos.—, —, —, —, and —.

The Sisters of No.— who had to leave their hospital at —— handed their sick officers and men over to the French hospital, much to their disgust. The officers especially have a horror of the elegant ways of the French nurses, who make one water do for washing them all round!

Tuesday, September 8th.

Orders came last night to each Matron to provide three or five Sisters who can talk French for duty up country with a Stationary Hospital, so M. and I are put down with two Regulars and another Reserve. It is probably too much luck and won't come off. The duties will be 'very strenuous', both for night and day duty, and we are to carry very little kit. The wire may come at any time. So this morning M. and I and Miss J——, our Senior Regular, and very nice indeed, got into the train for St Nazaire to see about our baggage, and had an adventurous morning. The place was swarming with troops of all sorts. The 6th Division was being sent up to the Front to-day, and no medical units could get hold of any transport for storing all their thousands of tons of stuff. One of the minor errors has been sending the 600 Sisters out with 600 trunks, 600 holdalls, and 600 kit-bags!! The Sisters' baggage is a byword now, and we could have done with only one of the three things or 1-1/2. We have been out nearly a month now and have not been near our boxes; some other hospitals have lost all theirs, or had them smashed up. We at last traced our No.— people and found them encamped on the wharf among the stuff, trying to get it stored with only one motor transport lent them by the Flying Corps. They were very nice to us, offered us lunch on packing-cases, and Major —— cleaned my skirt with petrol for me!

They sorted out the five kit-bags and boxes for us from the rest, as we have to go in to-morrow and repack for duty – only sleeping kit and uniform to be taken, and a change of underclothing. They said we'd have to make our own transport arrangements, as the 6th Division had taken up everything. So in the town we saw an empty dray outside a public-house, and after investigating inside two pubs we unearthed a fat man, who took us to a wine merchant's yard, and he produced a huge dray, which he handed over to us! We lent it to the Matron of No.—, and we have commandeered the brewer for No.—'s to-morrow. Then we met a large French motor ambulance without a French owner, with 'Havre' on it, which we knew, and sent Miss —— in it to the *Asturias* to try and collar it for us to-morrow. She did.

There were a lot of Cavalry already mounted just starting, and Welsh Fusiliers, and Argyll and Sutherlands, and swarms more. We had another invitation to a packing-case lunch from three other M.O.'s at another wharf, but couldn't stop.

We saw three German officers led through the crowd at the wharf. The French crowd booed and groaned and yelled 'Les Assassins' at them. The Tommies were quite quiet. They looked white and bored. We also saw 86 men (German prisoners) in a shed on the wharf. Some one who'd been talking to the

German officers told us they were quite cheerful and absolutely certain Germany is going to win!

Wednesday, September 9th.
It is a month to-day since I left home, and seems like six, and no work yet. Isn't it absolutely rotten? A big storm last night, and the Bay of Biscay tumbling about like fun to-day: bright and sunny again now. The French infants, boys and girls up to any age, are all dressed in navy knickers and jerseys and look so jolly. Matron has gone into St Nazaire to-day to get all the whole boiling of our baggage out here to repack. P'raps she'll bring some news or some letters, or, best of all, some orders.

This is a lovely spot. I'm writing on our balcony at the Riffelalp, above the tops of the pines, and straight over the sea. Three Padres are stranded at Pornichet – two were troopers in the S.A. War, and they do duty for us. The window of the glass lounge where we have services blew in with a crash this morning, right on the top of them, and it took some time to sort things out, but eventually they went on, in the middle of the sentence they stopped at.

A French rag this morning had some cheering telegrams about the Allies – that left, centre, and right were all more than holding their own, even if the enemy is rather near Paris. What about the Russians who came through England? We've heard of trains passing through Oxford with all the blinds down.

Thursday, September 10th.
Dazzling day. War news, 'L'ennemie se replie devant l'armée anglaise,' and that 'nos alliés anglais poursuivent leur offensive dans la direction de la Marne' – all good so far. No letters yet.

Friday, September 11th.
It is said to-day that No.— is to open at Nantes immediately. That will mean, at the earliest, in a fortnight, possibly much longer. We five French speakers are again told to stand by for special orders, but I know it won't come off.

At early service yesterday among the Intercessions was one

for patience in this time of trial waiting for our proper work. Never was there a more needful Intercession.

Some of us explored the salt-marshes behind this belt of pines yesterday, up to the farms and to a little old church on the other side; it was open, and had a little ship hanging over the chancel. The salt-marshes are intersected by sea walls – with sea pinks and sea lavender – that you walk along, and there are masses of blackberries round the farms.

There are rumours that all the hospitals will be getting to work soon, but I don't believe it. No.— has lost all its tent-poles, and a lot of its equipment in the move from Havre. I believe the missing stuff is supposed to be on its way to Jersey in the *Welshman* with the German prisoners.

Saturday, September 12th.
Rien à dire. Tous les jours même chose – on attend des ordres, ce qui ne viennent jamais.

Sunday, September 13th.
The hospitals seem to be showing faint signs of moving. No.— has gone to Versailles, and No.— to Nantes. No.— would have gone to Versailles if they hadn't had the bad luck to lose their tent-poles in the *Welshman*, and their pay-sheets and a few other important items.

Had to play the hymns at three services to-day without a hymn-book! Luckily I scratched up 370, 197, 193, 176, and 285, and 'God Save the King', out of my head, but 'We are but little children weak' is the only other I can do, except 'Peace, Perfect Peace'! A fine sermon by an exceptionally good Padre, mainly on Patience and Preparation!

Sunday Evening, September 13th, La Baule, Nantes.
Orders at last. M. and I, an Army Sister, and two Army Staff Nurses are to go to Le Mans; what for, remains to be seen; anyway, it will be work. It seems too good to be by any possibility true. We may be for Railway Station duty, feeding and dressings in trains or for a Stationary Hospital, or anything,

or to join No. 5 General at Le Mans.

Monday, September 14th, Angers, 8 p.m. – *in the train.*
We five got into the train at La Baule with kit-bags and holdalls, with the farewells of Matron and our friends, at 9.30 this morning. We are still in the same train, and shall not reach Le Mans till 11 p.m. Then what? Perhaps Station Duty, perhaps Hospital. There is said to be any amount of work at Le Mans. We have an R.H.A. Battery on this train with guns, horses, five officers, and trucks full of shouting and yelling men all very fit, straight from home. One big officer said savagely, 'The first man not carrying out orders will be sent down to the base,' to one of his juniors, as the worst threat. The spirits of the men are irrepressible. The French people rush up wherever we stop (which is extremely often and long) and give them grapes and pears and cigarettes. We have had cider, coffee, fruit, chocolate, and biscuits-and-cheese at intervals. It is difficult to get anything, because no one, French or English, ever seems to know when the train is going on.

We have been reading in *The Times* of September 3, 4, 5, and 7, all day, and re-reading last night's mail from home.

What a marvellous spirit has been growing in all ranks of the Army (and Navy) these last dozen years, to show as it is doing now. And the technical perfection of all one saw at the Military Tournament this year must have meant a good deal – for this War.

(We are still shunting madly in and out of Angers.)

Le Mans

WOUNDED FROM THE AISNE

September 15, 1914, to October 11, 1914

Station duty—On train duty—Orders again—Waiting to
go—Still at Le Mans—No.— Stationary Hospital—Off at
last—The Swindon of France.

Tuesday, September 15th.
The train managed to reach Le Mans at 1 a. m. this morning,
and kindly shunted into a siding in the station till 6.30 a. m.
so we got out our blankets and had a bit of a sleep. At 7 a
motor ambulance took us up to No.— Stationary Hospital,
which is a rather grimy Bishop's Palace, pretty full and busy.
The Sisters there gave us tea and biscuits, and we were then
sorted out by the Senior Matron, and billeted singly. I'm in a
nice little house with a garden with an old French lady who
hasn't a word of English, and fell on my neck when she found
I could understand her, and patter glibly and atrociously back.
My little room has a big window over the garden, and will,
I suppose, be my headquarters for the present in between
train and station duty, which I believe is to be our lot. We go
to a rather dim café for meals, and shall then learn what the
duty is to be. It is yet a long time coming. We haven't had a
meal since the day before yesterday, so I shall be glad when
12 o'clock comes. Now for a wash.

Wednesday, September 16th.

Still here: only four of the twenty-five (five sets of five) who formed our unit have been found jobs so far: two are taking a train of sick down to St Nazaire, and two have joined No.— Stationary Hospital in the town. We still await orders! This is a first-class War for awaiting orders for some of us.

Yesterday it poured all day. We explored the Cathedral, which is absolutely beautiful, perched high up over an open space – now crowded with transport and motor ambulances. We made tea in my quarters, and then explored the town; narrow streets thronged with Tommies as usual.

We have lunch at eleven and dinner at seven, at a dingy little inn through a smelly back yard; there is not much to eat, and you fill up with rather nasty bread and unripe pears, and drink a sort of flat cider, as the water is not good.

To-day it is sunny again. I have just been to High Mass (Choral), and taken photos of the Cathedral and the Market below, where I got four ripe peaches for 1-1/2d.

Writing in the garden of Mme. Bontevin, my landlady.

There is any amount of work here at the Bishop's Palace; more than they can get through on night duty with bad cases, and another Jesuit College has been opened as No.— Stationary. Went up to No.— S. this afternoon where F—— has been sent, to see her; she asked me to go out and buy cakes for six wounded officers. They seemed highly pleased with them; they are on beds, the men on stretchers; all in holland sheets and brown blankets; only bare necessaries, as the Stationary Hospitals have to be very mobile: stretchers make very decent beds, but they are difficult for nursing.

They have had a good many deaths, surgical and medical, at L'Evêché; they have pneumonias, and paralysis, and septic wounds, and an officer shot through the head, with a temperature of 106 and paralysis; there is a civil surgeon with a leg for amputation at No.— Stationary.

Friday, September 18th.

Même chose. We go up to the Hospital and ask for orders, and

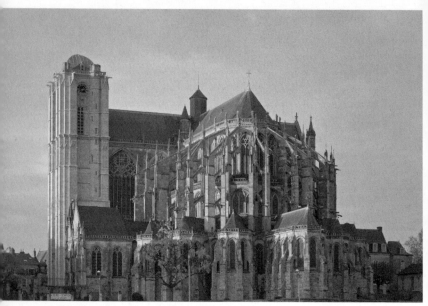

The cathedral at Le Mans.

to-night we were both told to get into ward uniform in the morning, and wait there in case a job turns up. I've just come to-night from No.— Station where F—— is, to take her some things she asked me to get for her officers.

They have been busy at the station to-day doing dressings on the trains. A lot have come down from this fighting on the Marne.

Yesterday I think one touched the bottom of this waiting business. The food at the dingy inn has dérangé my inside, and I lay down all day yesterday. The Sergeant at the Dispensary prescribed lead and opium pills for me when I asked for chlorodyne, as he said he'd just cured a General with the same complaint—from the sour bread, he said. Fanny, the fat cook here, and Isabel the maid, were overcome with anxiety over my troubles, and fell over each other with hot bottles, and drinks, and advice. They are perfect angels. Madame Bontevin pays me a state call once a day; she has to have all the windows shut, and we sit close and converse with animation. Flowery

French compliments simply fly between us. We often have to help the Tommies out with their shopping; their attempts to buy Beecham's Pills are the funniest.

This afternoon I found *The Times* of September 15th (Tuesday of this week) in a shop and had a happy time with it. It referred, in a Frenchman's letter, to a sunset at Havre on an evening that he would never forget – nor shall I – with an American cruiser and a troopship going out. (See page 24 of this effusion.)

Saturday, September 19th.
It seems that we five No.—s who came up last Monday are being kept to staff another Stationary Hospital farther up, when it is ready; at least that is what it looks like from sundry rumours – if so – good enough.

We have been all day in caps and aprons at L'Evêché, marking linen and waiting for orders on the big staircase. I've also been over both hospitals. The bad cases all seem to be dropped here off the trains; there are some awful mouth, jaw, head, leg, and spine cases, who can't recover, or will only be crippled wrecks. You can't realise that it has all been done on purpose, and that none of them are accidents or surgical diseases. And they seem all to take it as a matter of course; the bad ones who are conscious don't speak, and the better ones are all jolly and smiling, and ready 'to have another smack'. One little room had two wounded German prisoners, with an armed guard. One who was shot through the spine died while I was there – his orderly and the Sister were with him. The other is a spy – nearly well – who has to be very carefully watched.

They are all a long time between the field and the Hospital. One told me he was wounded on Tuesday – was one day in a hospital, and then travelling till to-day, Saturday. No wonder their wounds are full of straw and grass. (Haven't heard of any more tetanus.) Most haven't had their clothes off, or washed, for three weeks, except face and hands.

No war news to-day, except that the Germans are well fortified and entrenched in their positions N. of Rheims.

Sunday, September 20th.

Began with early service at the Jesuit School Hospital at 6.30, and the rest of the day one will never forget. The fighting for these concrete entrenched positions of the Germans behind Rheims has been so terrific since last Sunday that the number of casualties has been enormous. Three trains full of wounded, numbering altogether 1175 cases, have been dressed at the station to-day; we were sent down at 11 this morning. The train I was put to had 510 cases. You boarded a cattle-truck, armed with a tray of dressings and a pail; the men were lying on straw; had been in trains for several days; most had only been dressed once, and many were gangrenous. If you found one urgently needed amputation or operation, or was likely to die, you called an M.O. to have him taken off the train for Hospital. No one grumbled or made any fuss. Then you joined the throng in the dressing-station, and for hours doctors of all ranks, Sisters and orderlies, grappled with the stream of stretchers, and limping, staggering, bearded, dirty, fagged men, and ticketed them off for the motor ambulances to the Hospitals, or back to the train, after dressing them. The platform was soon packed with stretchers with all the bad cases waiting patiently to be taken to Hospital. We cut off the silk vest of a dirty, brigandish-looking officer, nearly finished with a wound through his lung. The Black Watch and Camerons were almost unrecognisable in their rags. The staple dressing is tincture of iodine; you don't attempt anything but swabbing with lysol, and then gauze dipped in iodine. They were nearly all shrapnel shell wounds—more ghastly than anything I have ever seen or smelt; the Mauser wounds of the Boer War were pin-pricks compared with them. There was also a huge train of French wounded being dressed on the other side of the station, including lots of weird, gaily-bedecked Zouaves.

There was no real confusion about the whole day, owing to the good organising of the No.— Clearing Hospital people who run it. Every man was fed, and dressed and sorted. They'll have a heavy time at the two hospitals to-night with the cases sent up from the trains.

M. and I are now – 9 p.m. – in charge of a train of 141 (with an M.O. and two orderlies) for St Nazaire; we jump out at the stations and see to them, and the orderlies and the people on the stations feed them: we have the worst cases next to us. We may get there some time to-morrow morning, and when they are taken off, we train back, arriving probably on Wednesday at Le Mans. The lot on this train are the best leavings of to-day's trains, – a marvellously cheery lot, munching bread and jam and their small share of hot tea, and blankets have just been issued. We ourselves have a rug, and a ration of bread, tea, and jam; we had dinner on the station.

When I think of your Red Cross practices on boy scouts, and the grim reality, it makes one wonder. And the biggest wonder of it all is the grit there is in them, and the price they are individually and unquestioningly paying for doing their bit in this War.

Monday, September 21st.
In train on way back to Le Mans from St Nazaire. We did the journey in twelve hours, and arrived at 9 this morning, which was very good, considering the congestion on the line. In the middle of the night we pulled up alongside an immense troop train, taking a whole Brigade of D. of Cornwall's L.I. up to the front, such a contrast to our load coming away from the front. Our lot will be a long time getting to bed; the Medical Officers at St N. told us there were already two trains in, and no beds left on hospitals or ships, and 1300 more expected to-day; four died in one of the trains; ours were pretty well, after the indescribable filth and fug of the train all night; it was not an ambulance train, but trucks and ordinary carriages. The men say there are hardly any officers left in many regiments. There has never been this kind of rush to be coped with anywhere, but the Germans must be having worse. We had thirteen German prisoners tacked on to us with a guard of the London Scottish, the first Territorials to come out, bursting with health and pride and keenness. They are not in the fighting line yet, but are used as escorts for the G.P. among other jobs. One of the men on

our train had had his shoulder laid open for six inches by a shell, where he couldn't see the wound. He asked me if it was a bullet wound! He himself thought it was too large for that, and might be shrapnel! He hadn't mentioned it all night.

We had some dressings to be done again this morning, and then left them in charge of the M.O. and two orderlies, and went to report ourselves to the A.D.M.S. and get a warrant for the return journey. We shall get in to Le Mans somewhere about midnight. I'm not a bit tired, strange to say; we got a few rests in the night, but couldn't sleep.

Tuesday, September 22nd.

Got back to Le Mans at 2 a.m.– motor-ambulanced up to the hospital, where an orderly made lovely beds for us on stretchers, with brown blankets and pillows, in the theatre, and labelled the door 'Operation', in case anyone should disturb us. At 6 we went to our respective diggings for a wash and breakfast, and reported to Matron at 8. We have been two days and two nights in our clothes; food where, when, and what one could get; one wash only on a station platform at a tap which a sergeant kindly pressed for me while I washed! One cleaning of teeth in the dark on the line between trucks. They have no water on trains or at stations, except on the engine, which makes tea in cans for you for the men when it stops.

We are to rest to-day, to be ready for another train to-night if necessary. The line from the front to Rouen – where there are two General Hospitals – is cut; hence this appalling over-crowding at our base. When we got back this morning, nine of those we took off the trains on Sunday afternoon had died here, and one before he reached the hospital – three of tetanus. I haven't heard how many at the other hospital at the Jesuit school – tetanus there too. Some of the amputations die of septic absorption and shock, and you wouldn't wonder if you saw them. I went to the 9 o'clock Choral High Mass this morning at that glorious and beautiful Cathedral – all gorgeous old glass and white and grey stone, slender Gothic and fat Norman. It was very fine and comforting.

The sick officers are frightfully pleased to see *The Times*, no matter how old; so are we. I've asked M. to collect their 1/2*d*. picture daily papers once a week for the men.

Wednesday, September 23rd.
Have been helping in the wards at No.— to-day. The Sisters and orderlies there have all about twice what they can get through – the big dressings are so appalling and new cases have been coming in – all stretcher cases. As soon as they begin to recover at all they are sent down to the base to make room for worse ones off the trains. To-morrow I am on station duty again – possibly for another train.

There is a rumour that three British cruisers have been sunk by a submarine – it can't be true.

I don't see why this battle along the French frontier should ever come to an end, at any rate till both armies are exhausted, and decide to go to bed. The men say we can't spot their guns – they are too well hidden in these concrete entrenchments.

The weather is absolutely glorious all day, and the stars all night. Orion, with his shining bodyguard, from Sirius to Capella, is blazing every morning at 4.

Thursday, September 24th, 3 p.m.
Taking 480 sick and wounded down to St Nazaire, with a junior staff nurse, one M.O., and two orderlies. Just been feeding them all at Angers; it is a stupendous business. The train is miles long – not corridor or ambulance; they have straw to lie on the floors and stretchers. The M.O. has been two nights in the train already on his way down from the front (four miles from the guns), and we joined on to him with a lot of hospital cases sent down to the base. I've been collecting the worst ones into carriages near ours all the way down when we stop; but of course you miss a good many. Got my haversack lined with jaconet and filled with cut-dressings, very convenient, as you have both hands free. We continually stop at little stations, so you can get to a good many of them, and we get quite expert at clawing along the footboards; some of the men, with their

eyes, noses, or jaws shattered, are so extraordinarily good and uncomplaining. Got hold of a spout-feeder and some tubing at Angers for a boy in the Grenadier Guards, with a gaping hole through his mouth to his chin, who can't eat, and cannot otherwise drink. The French people bring coffee, fruit, and all sorts of things to them when we stop.

We shall have to wait at St Nazaire all day, and come back by night to-morrow.

One swanky Ambulance Train carries four permanent Sisters to the front to fetch cases to Le Mans and the Base. They go to Villeneuve. They say the country is deserted, crops left to waste, houses empty, and when you get there no one smiles or speaks, but listens to the guns. The men seem to think the Germans have got our range, but we haven't found theirs. The number of casualties must be nearly into five figures this last battle alone; and when you think of the Russians, the Germans, the French, the Austrians, and the Belgians all like that, the whole convulsion seems more meaningless than ever for civilised nations.

This is in scraps, owing to the calls of duty. The beggars simply swarm out of the train at every stop – if they can limp or pull up by one arm – to get the fruit and things from the French.

Friday, September 25th.
In train back to Le Mans, 9 p.m. We landed our tired, stiff, painful convoy at St Nazaire at 8.45 yesterday evening. The M.O.'s there told us our lot made 1800 that had come down since early morning; one load of bad cases took eight hours to unload. The officers all seemed depressed and overworked, and they were having a very tight fit to get beds for them at the various hospitals at St Nazaire. At about 10 p.m. the last were taken off by the motor ambulances, and we got some dinner on the station with our Civil Surgeon, who was looking forward to a night in a tent out of a train.

The R.T.O. found us an empty 1st class carriage in the station to sleep in, and the sergeant found us a candle and matches and put us to bed, after a sketchy wash provided by the buffet lady.

The din was continuous all night, so one didn't sleep much, but had a decent rest (and a flea). The sergeant called us at 6.30, and we had another sketchy wash, and coffee and rolls and jam at the buffet. Then we found our way to the hospital ship *Carisbrook Castle*. The Army Sister in charge was most awfully kind, showed us over, made the steward turn on hot baths for us, provided notepaper, kept us to lunch – the nicest meal we've seen for weeks! The ship had 500 cases on board, and was taking 200 more – many wounded officers.

A captain of the —— told me all his adventures from the moment he was hit till now. His regiment had nine officers killed and twenty-seven wounded. He said they knew things weren't going well in that retreat, but they never knew how critical it was at the time.

After lunch, we took our grateful leave and went to the A.D.M.S.'s office for our return warrants for the R.T.O. (I have just had to sign it for fourteen, as senior officer of our two selves and twelve A.S.C. men taking two trucks of stores, who have no officer with them!) There we heard that ten of our No.— Sisters were ordered to Nantes for duty by the 4.28, so we hied back to the station to meet them and see them off. They were all frightfully glad to be on the move at last, and we had a great meeting. The rest are still bathing at La Baule and cursing their luck.

While we were getting some coffee in the only *patisserie* in the dirty little town, seven burly officer boys of the Black Watch came in to buy cakes for the train, they said, to-night. They were nearly all second lieutenants, one captain, and were so excited at going up to the Front they couldn't keep still. They asked us eagerly if we'd had many of 'our regiment' wounded, and how many casualties were there, and how was the fighting going, and how long would the journey take. (The nearer you get to the Front the longer it takes, as trains are always having to shunt and go round loops to make room for supply trains.) They didn't seem to have the dimmest idea what they're in for, bless them. They are on this train in the next carriage.

The Padre told me he was the only one at St Nazaire for all the hospitals and all the troops in camp (15,000 in one camp alone).

He had commandeered the Bishop of Khartoum to help him, and another bishop, who both happen to be here.

We are now going to turn out the light, and hope for the best till they come to look at the warrant or turn us out to change.

6 a.m.– At Sablé at 4 a.m. we were turned out for two hours; a wee open station. Mr —— and our Civil Surgeon were most awfully decent to us: turned a sleepy official out of a room for us, and at 5 came and dug us out to have coffee and *brioches* with them. Then we went for a sunrise walk round the village, and were finally dragged into their carriage, as they thought it was more comfortable than ours. Just passed a big French ambulance train full from Compiègne.

At Le Mans the train broke up again, and everybody got out. We motor-ambulanced up to the Hospital with the three night Sisters coming off station duty. Matron wanted us to go to bed for the day; but we asked to come on after lunch, as they were busy and we weren't overtired. I'm realising to-night that I have been on the train four nights out of six, and bed is bliss at this moment.

I was sent to No.— Stationary at the Jesuits' College to take over the officers at one o'clock.

One was an angelic gunner boy with a septic leg and an undaunted smile, except when I dressed his leg and he said, 'Oh, damn!' The other bad one was wounded in the shoulder. They kept me busy till Sister —— came back, and then I went to my beloved Cathedral (and vergered some Highland Tommies round it, they had fits of awe and joy over it, and grieved over 'Reems'). It is awfully hard to make these sick officers comfortable, with no sheets or pillow-cases, no air ring-cushions, pricky shirts, thick cups without saucers, etc. One longs for the medical comforts of ——

I hear to-night that Miss ——, the Principal Matron on the

Lines of Communication (on the War Establishment Staff) is here again, and may have a new destination for some of us details.

The heading in 'Le Matin' to-night is:—

UNE LUTTE ACHARNÉE
DE LA SOMME A LA MEUSE
LA BATAILLE REDOUBLE DE VIOLENCE

If it redoubles *de violence* much longer who will be left?

Sunday, September 27th.
My luck is in this time. Miss —— has just sent for me to tell me I am for permanent duty on No.— Ambulance Train (equipped) which goes up to the Front, to the nearest point on the rail to the fighting line. Did you ever know such luck? There are four of us, one Army Sister and me and two juniors; we live altogether on the train. The train will always be pushed up as near the Field Hospitals as the line gets to, whether we drive the Germans back to Berlin or they drive us into the sea. It is now going to Braisne, a little east of Soissons, just S. of the Aisne, N.E. of Rheims. It is on its way up now, and we are to join it with our baggage when it stops here on the way to St Nazaire. We shall have two days and two nights with wounded, and two days and two nights to rest on the return empty. The work itself will be of the grimmest possible, as we shall have all the worst cases, being an equipped Hospital in a train. It was worth waiting five weeks to get this; every man or woman stuck at the Base has dreams of getting to the Front, but only one in a hundred gets the dream fulfilled.

There is no doubt that 'the horrors of War' have outdone themselves by this modern perfection of machinery killing, and the numbers involved, as they have never done before, and as it was known they would. The details are often unprintable. They have eight cases of tetanus at No.— Stationary, and five have died.

All the patients at No.— have been inoculated against tetanus to-day. They have it in the French Hospitals too.

Went to the Voluntary Evening Service for the troops at the theatre at 5. The Padres and a Union Jack and the Allies' Flags; and a piano on the stage; officers and sisters in the stalls; and the rest packed tight with men: they were very reverent, and nearly took the roof off in the Hymns, Creed, and Lord's Prayer. Excellent sermon. We had the War Intercessions and a good prayer I didn't know, ending with 'Strengthen us in life, and comfort us in death'. The men looked what they were, British to the bone; no one could take them for any other nation a mile off. Clean, straight, thin, sunburnt, clear-eyed, all at their Active Service best, no pallid rolls of fat on their faces like the French. The man who preached must have liked talking to them in that pin-dropped silence and attention; he evidently knows his opportunities.

Monday, September 28th.
There are hundreds of people in deep new black in this town; what must it be in Berlin? The cemetery here is getting full of French and British soldiers' graves. Those 1200 sailors from the three cruisers had fine clean quick deaths compared to what happens here.

We have got our baggage (kit-bags and holdalls) down to the station at the Red Cross Anglaise, and are sitting in our quarters waiting for the word to come that No.— train is in. Met Miss —— in her car in the town, and she said that it was just possible that the train might go down to Havre this journey, she wasn't dead sure it was doing this route! If so we shall be nicely and completely sold, as I don't know how we should ever join it. But I'm not going to believe in such bad luck as that would be till it happens.

Tuesday, September 29th.
We *were* sold last night after all. Trailed down to the station to await the train according to orders, and were then told by the A.D.M.S. that it had gone to Havre this journey, and couldn't be on this line till next week, and we could go to bed. So after

all the embraces of Mme. and Fanny and Isabel, I turned up at 10.30 to ask for a bed. 'Ma pauvre demoiselle,' said fat F., hastening to let me in.

This morning Miss —— came down with us to the A.D.M.S.'s Office to find out how we could join the train, and he said: 'Wait till it comes in next week, and meanwhile go on duty at the Hospital.' I don't mind anything as long as we do eventually get on to the train, and we are to do that, so one must possess one's soul in patience. I am back with the sick officers at No.— Stationary.

There are rumours to-night of bad news from the front, and that the German Navy is emerging from Kiel.

Wednesday, September 30th.
Have been doing the sick officers all day (or rather wounded). They are quite nice, but the lack of equipment makes twice the work. We are still having bright sunny days, but it is getting cold, and I shall be glad of warmer clothes. The food at the still filthy Inn in a dark outhouse through the back yard has improved a little! My Madame (in my billet) gives me coffee and bread and butter (of the best) at 7, and there is a ration tin of jam, and I have acquired a pot of honey.

On duty at 7.30 a.m.– At 12 or 1 we go to the Inn for *déjeûner*: meat of some sort, one vegetable, bread, butter, and cheese, and pears. Tea we provide ourselves when we can.

At 7 or 8 we go to the Inn and have *potage* (which is warm water with a few stray onions or carrots in it), and tough cold meat, and sometimes a piece of pastry (for pudding), bread, butter, and cheese, and a very small cup of coffee, and little, rather hard pears. I am very well on it now since they changed the bread, though pretty tired.

Thursday, October 1st.
The sky in Mid France on October 1st is of a blue that outblues the bluest that June or any other month can do in l'Angleterre. It is cold in the early mornings and evenings, dazzling all day, and shining moon by night.

The H.A.C. are all over the town: they do orderly duty at Headquarters and all the Offices; they seem to be gentlemen in Tommy's kit; fine big lot they are. Taking it all round, the Regular British Army on Active Service – from hoary, beribboned Generals, decorated Staff Officers of all ranks, other officers, and N.C.O.'s down to the humblest Tommy – is the politest and best-mannered thing I have ever met, with few exceptions. Wherever you are, or go, or have to wait, they come and ask if they can do anything for you, generally with an engaging smile seize your hand-baggage, offer you chairs and see you through generally. And the men and N.C.O.'s are just the same, and always awfully grateful if you can help them out with the language in any way.

This was a conversation I heard in my ward to-day. Brother of Captain —— (wounded) visits the amputation man, and, by way of cheering him up, sits down, gazes at his ugly bandaged stump on a pillow, and says –

'That must be the devil.'

'Yes, it is,' says the leg man.

'Hell,' says the other, and then they both seemed to feel better and began to talk of something else.

We had a funeral of an Orderly and a German from No.— Sta. (both tetanus). On grey transport waggons with big black horses, wreaths from the Orderlies, carried by a big R.A.M.C. escort (which, of course, escorted the German too), with Officers and Padre and two Sisters.

Friday, October 2nd.

They continue to die every day and night at both Hospitals, though we are taking few new cases in now.

I am frightfully attached to Le Mans as a place. The town is old and curly, and full of lovely corners and 'Places', and views and Avenues and Gardens. The Cathedral grows more and more upon one; I have several special spots where you get the most exquisite poems of colour and stone, where I go and browse; it is very quiet and beautifully kept.

No.— Sta. is also set in a jewel of a spot. A Jesuits' College, full of cloisters covered with vines, and lawns with silver statues, shady avenues and sunny gardens, long corridors and big halls which are the wards; the cook-house is a camp under a splendid row of big chestnut trees, and there is of course a chapel.

Our occupation of it is rather incongruous; there is practically no furniture except the boys' beds, some chairs, many crucifixes and statues, terribly primitive sanitary arrangements and water supply. We have to boil our instruments and make their tea in the same one saucepan in the Officers' Ward; you do without dusters, dishcloths, soap-dishes, pillow-cases, and many other necessities in peace time.

My little Train-Junior has been taken off that job and is to rejoin her unit, so I settled down to a prospect of the same fate (No.— G.H. is at Havre again! and has still not yet done any work! so you see what I've been rescued from). I met Miss —— to-night and asked her, and she says I *am* going on the train when it comes in, so I breathe again.

Tuesday, October 6th.

I am now dividing my time between the top floor of Tommies and five Germans and the Officers' Ward, where I relieve S. —— — for meals and off duty. There are some bad dressings in the top ward. The five Germans are quiet, fat, and amenable, glad to exchange a few remarks in their own language. I haven't had time to try and talk to them, but will if I can; two of them are very badly wounded. Some of the medical Tommies make the most of very small ailments, but the surgicals are wonderful boys.

Wednesday, October 7th.

I have been down to the station this evening; heard that St Nazaire is being given up as a base, which means that no more ambulance trains will come through.

The five Germans in my ward told me this morning that only the Reichstag and the Kaiser wanted the War; that Russia began it, so Deutschland *mussen*; that Deutschland couldn't win against Russia, France, England, Belgium, and Japan; and that there were no more men in Germany to replace the killed. They smiled peacefully at the prospect and said it was *ganz gut* to be going to England. They have fat, pink, ruminating, innocent, fair faces, and are very obedient. I made one of them scrub the floor, as the Orderly had a bad arm from inoculation, and he seemed to enjoy it. Only one is married.

Thursday, October 8th.
There was a very picturesque and rather touching scene at No.— this afternoon. They had a concert in the open quadrangle, with vined cloisters on all four sides, and holy statues and crucifixes about. In the middle were the audience – rows of stretchers with contented Tommies smoking and enjoying it (some up in their grey-blue pyjamas), and many Orderlies, some Sisters and M.O.'s and French priests; the piano on a platform at one end.

Friday, October 9th.
My compound fractured femur man told me how he stopped his bullet. Some wounded Germans held up the white flag and he went to them to help them. When he was within seven yards, the man he was going to help shot him in the thigh. A Coldstream Guardsman with him then split the German's head open with the butt-end of his rifle. The wounded Tommy was eventually taken to the château of the 'lidy what killed the Editor somewhere in this country.'

Saturday, October 10th.
'Orders by Lt.-Col. ——, R.A.M.C., A.D.M.S., Advanced Base Headquarters, October 10th, 1914. Sister —— will proceed to Villeneuve Triage to-day, and on arrival will report to Major ——, R.A.M.C, for duty on Ambulance Trains.'

So it's come at last, and I have handed over my officers, and am now installed by the R.T.O. in a 1st class carriage to myself with all my kit, and my lovely coat and muffler, and rug and cushion, after a pleasant dinner of tea, cheese, and ration biscuits in the Red Cross Dressing Room, with a kind Army Sister.

The R.T.O. this time has given me (instead of 12 A.S.C. men) a highly important envelope marked Very Urgent, to give to the Director of Supplies, Villeneuve, whoever he is.

Change at Versailles in about six hours, so I may as well try and get some sleep.

I was really sorry to say good-bye to my kind old Madame Bontevin, 22 Rue de la Motte, and fat Fanny, and charming Isabel, and my nice little room – (a heavenly bed!) – and ducky little gay garden, where I've lived for the last month; and my beloved Cathedral, and lots of the Sisters I have got to know.

Versailles, 7 a.m. *Sunday, October 11th.*
At 3 a.m. at Chartres an officer of a Zouave Regiment, in blue and gold Zouave, blue sash, crimson bags like petticoats, and black puttees, and his smartly dressed sister, came into my carriage; both very nice and polite and friendly. He was 21, had fought in three campaigns, and been wounded twice; now convalescent after a wound in the foot a month ago – going to the depôt to rejoin. Her husband also at the front, and another brother. I changed at Versailles, and was given tea, and a slight wash by the always hospitable station duty Sisters, who welcome you at every big station. The No.— G.H. here they belong to is a very fine hotel with lovely gardens, and they are very proud of it – close to the Palace.

10 a.m. *Juvisy.* I am now in an empty 1st class saloon (where I can take a long walk) after a long wait, with *café au lait* and an omelette at Juvisy, and *The Times* of October 5th.

There is a pleasing uncertainty about one's own share on Active Service. I haven't the slightest idea whether, when I get to Villeneuve in half an hour's time, I shall

(*a*) Remain there awaiting orders either in a French billet, a railway carriage, or a tent;

(*b*) Be sent up to Braisne to join a train; or

(*c*) Be sent down to Havre to ditto.

We had a man in No.— Stationary who got through the famous charge of the 9th Lancers unhurt, but came into hospital for an ingrowing toe nail!

Villeneuve, 5 p.m. Like a blithering idiot, I was so interested in the Gunner's Diary of his birthday 'in my hole' that I passed Villeneuve Triage, and got out the station after! Had to wait 1-1/2 hours for a train back, and got here eventually at 12. Collared four polite London Scottish to carry my baggage, and found the Sister in charge of Train Ambulance people.

I wish I could describe this extraordinary place. It is the Swindon of France; a huge wilderness of railway lines, trains, and enormous hangars, now used as camps and hospitals. Sister B. is encamped in a shut-off corner of one of these sheds surrounded by London Scottish cooking and making tea in little groups; they swarm here. I sleep to-night in the same small bed in an empty cottage with a Sister I've never seen before. We meal at a Convent French Hospital. I delivered my 'Very Urgent' envelope to the R.T.O. for the Director of Supplies, and reported to Major ——, and after lunch had an hour's sleep on The Bed. There are rows of enterics on stretchers in khaki in this shed, waiting for motor ambulances to take them to Versailles No.— G.H., being nursed here meanwhile. There are also British prisoners (defaulters) penned in in another corner, and French troops at the other end!

On No.— Ambulance Train (1)

FIRST EXPERIENCES

October 13, 1914, to October 19, 1914.

Ambulance Train—Under fire—Tales of the Retreat—Life on
the Train.

Tuesday, October 13th.
At last I am on the train, and have just unpacked. There is an
Army Sister and two Reserve, a Major ——, O.C., and two
junior officers.

Don't know yet what messing arrangements are. We each
have a bunk to ourselves, with a proper mattress, pillow, and
blankets: a table and seat at one end, lots of racks and hooks,
and a lovely little washing-house leading out of the bunk, shared
by the two Sisters on each side of it: each has a door into it. No
one knows where we are going; we start this afternoon.

6 p.m. Not off yet. We had lunch in a small dining-car, we
four Sisters at one table, Major —— and his two Civil Surgeons
at another, and some French officials of the train at another.
Meal cooked and served by the French – quite nice, no cloth,
only one knife and fork. They are all very friendly and jolly.

In between the actual dealing with the wounded, which is only
too real, it all feels like a play or a dream: why should the whole
of France, at any rate along the railways and places on them, be
upside down, swarming with British soldiers, and all, French and

English, working for and talking of the one thing? Everything, and every house and every hotel, school, and college, being used for something different from what it was meant for; the billeting is universal. You hear a funny alternation of educated and uneducated English on all sides of you, and loud French gabbling of all sorts. By day you see aeroplanes and troop trains and artillery trains; and by night you see searchlights and hear the incessant wailing and squawking of the train whistles. On every platform and at every public doors or gates are the red and blue French soldiers with their long spikey bayonets, or our Tommies with the short broad bayonets that don't look half so deadly though I expect they are much worse. You either have to have a written passport up here, or you must know the 'mot' if challenged by the French sentries. All this from Havre and St Nazaire up to the Front.

The train is one-third mile long, so three walks along its side gives you exercise for a mile. The ward beds are lovely: broad and soft, with lovely pillow-cases and soft thick blankets; any amount of dressings and surgical equipment, and a big kitchen, steward's store, and three orderlies to each waggon. Shouldn't be surprised if we get 'there' in the dark, and won't see the war country. Sometimes you are stopped by bridges being blown up in front of you, and little obstacles of that kind.

Wednesday, October 14th.

Still in the siding 'waiting for orders' to move on. There's a lot of waiting being done in this war one way and another, as well as a lot of doing. What a splendid message the French Government have sent the Belgian Government on coming to Havre! exciting for the people at Havre: they used to go mad when dusty motor-cars with a few exhausted-looking Belgians arrived in Havre.

We seem to be going to Rouen and up from there. Villeneuve is going to be evacuated as a military P.O. centre and other headquarters, and Abbeville to be the place – west of Amiens.

I had an excellent night, no sheets (because of the difficulties of washing), my own rug next me, and lots of blankets: the

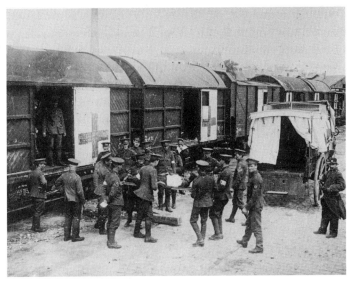

A Red Cross ambulance train.

view, with trucks on each side, is not inspiring, but will improve when we move: have only been allowed walks alongside the train to-day because it may move at any minute (although it has no engine as yet!), and you mayn't leave the train without a pass from the Major.

M.O.'s and Sisters live on one waggon, all our little doors opening into the same corridor, where we have tea; it is a very easy family party. Our beds are all sofas in the daytime and quite public, unless we like to shut our doors. It is pouring to-day – first wet day for weeks.

Orders just come that we move at 8.46 for Abbeville, and get orders for the Front from there.

6.30 p.m. Another order just come that our destination is Braisne, not Abbeville. They have always seen shells bursting at Braisne. I'm glad it's Braisne, as we shall get to the other part next journey, I expect.

8.45 p.m. Started at last.

Thursday, October 15th, 10 a.m.

Braisne. Got here about 8 o'clock. After daylight only evidence of the war I could see from my bed were long lines of French troops in the roads, and a few British camps; villages all look deserted. Guns booming in the distance, sounds like heavy portmanteaux being dropped on the roof at regular intervals. Some London Scottish on the station say all the troops have gone from here except themselves and the R.A.M.C. There are some wounded to come on here.

There is an R.E. camp just opposite in a very wet wood, and quagmires of mud. They have built Kaffir kraals to sleep in – very sodden-looking; they've just asked for some papers; we had a few. They build pontoons over the Aisne at night and camp here by day.

4 p.m. We have only taken twelve cases on as yet, but are having quite an exciting afternoon. Shells are coming at intervals into the village. I've seen two burst in the houses, and one came right over our train. Two French soldiers on the line lay flat on their faces; one or two orderlies got under the train; one went on fishing in the pond close by, and the wounded Tommies got rather excited, and translated the different sounds of 'them Jack Johnsons' and 'them Coal-boxes' and 'Calamity Kate', and of our guns and a machine-gun popping. There is a troop train just behind us that they may be potting at, or some gunners in the village, or the R.E. camp. There have been two aeroplanes over us this afternoon. You hear the shell coming a long way off, rather like a falsetto motor-engine, and then it bursts (twice in the trees of this wood where we are standing). There is an endless line of French horse transport winding up the wood on the other side, and now some French cavalry. The R.T.O. is now having the train moved to a safer place.

The troops have all gone except the 1st Division, who are waiting for the French to take their place, and then all the British will be on the Arras line, I believe, where we shall go next. (There's another close to the train.) They make such a fascinating purring noise coming, ending in a singing scream;

you have to jump up and see. It is a yellowish-green sound! But you can't see it till it bursts.

None of the twelve taken on need any looking after at night besides what the orderly can do, so we shall go to bed.

We had another shell over the train, which (not the train) exploded with a loud bang in the wood the other side; made one jump more than any yet, and that was in the 'safer place' the R.T.O. had the train moved to.

Friday, October 16th, 2 p.m.

Have had a very busy time since last entry. The shelling of the village was aimed at the church, the steeple of which was being used by the French for signalling. A butcher was killed and a boy injured, and as the British Clearing Hospital was in the church and the French Hospital next door they were all cleared out into our train; many very bad cases, fractured spine, a nearly dying lung case, a boy with wound in lung and liver, three pneumonias, some bad enterics (though the worst have not been moved). A great sensation was having four badly wounded French women, one minus an arm, aged 16; another minus a foot, aged 61, amputation after shell wounds from a place higher up. They are in the compartment next three wounded officers. They are all four angelically good and brave and grateful; it does seem hard luck on them. It was not easy getting them all settled in, in a pitch-dark evening, the trains so high from the ground; and a good deal of excitement all round over the shelling, which only left off at dusk. One of the C.S.'s had a narrow shave on his way from the train to the R.T.O.; he had just time to lie flat, and it burst a few yards from him, on the line. S. and I stayed up till 3 a.m. and then called the others, and we got up again at 8 and were all busy all the morning. It is a weird business at night, picking your way through kitchens and storerooms and wards with a lantern over the rickety bridges and innumerable heavy swing-doors. I was glad of the brown overall G. sent me, and am wearing the mackintosh apron to-day that N. made me. We are probably staying here several days, and are doing day and night duty entire – not divided as last night. I am on day.

We have a great many washings in the morning, and have to make one water do for one compartment – (the train ran out of water this morning – since refilled from the river alongside); and bed-makings, and a lot of four-hourly treatment with the acutes. The enteric ward has a very good orderly, and excellent disinfecting arrangements. It is in my division of the train. Lack of drinking water makes things very difficult.

I thought things were difficult in the hospitals at Le Mans owing to lack of equipment, but that was child's play compared to the structural difficulties of working a hospital on a train, especially when it stands in a siding several days. One man will have to die on the train if we don't move soon, but we are not full up yet. Twenty-seven men – minor cases – bolted from the church yesterday evening on to the train when the shells were dropping, and were ignominiously sent back this morning.

It has so far been the most exciting journey the train has had. Jack Johnson has been very quiet all the morning, but he spoke for a little again just now. I'm going to have a rest now till four.

Four Tommies in one bunk yesterday told me things about the trenches and the fighting line, which you have to believe because they are obviously giving recent intimate personal experiences; but how do they or any one ever live through it? These came all through the Retreat from Mons. Then through the wet weather in the trenches on the Aisne – where they don't always get hot tea (as is said in the papers, much to their scorn). They even had to take the tea and sugar out of the haversacks of dead Germans; no one had had time to bury for twelve days – 'It warn't no use to them,' they said, 'and we could do with it.'

In the Retreat they said men's boots were worn right off and they marched without; the packs were thrown away, and the young boys died of exhaustion and heat. The officers guarded each pump in case they should drink bad water, and they drank water wrung out of their towels!

'And just as Bill got to the pump the shell burst on him – it made a proper mess of him' – this with a stare of horror. And they never criticise or rant about it, but accept it as their share for the time being.

The train is to-day in a place with a perfect wood on both sides, glowing with autumn colours, and through it goes a road with continual little parties of French cavalry, motors, and transport waggons passing up it.

Saturday, October 17th.
We are to stay here till Monday, to go on taking up the wounded from the 1st Division. They went on coming in all yesterday in motor ambulances. They come straight from the trenches, and are awfully happy on the train with the first attempts at comforts they have known. One told me they were just getting their tea one day, relieving the trenches, when 'one o' them coal-boxes' sent a 256 lb. shell into them, which killed seven and wounded fifteen. *One* shell! He said he had to help pick them up and it made him sick.

10 p.m. Wrote the last before breakfast, and we haven't sat down since. We are to move back to Villeneuve to-morrow, dropping the sick probably at Versailles. Every one thankful to be going to move at last. The gas has given out, and the entire train is lit by candles.

Imagine a hospital as big as King's College Hospital all packed into a train, and having to be self-provisioned, watered, sanitated, lit, cleaned, doctored and nursed and staffed and officered, all within its own limits. No outside person can realise the difficulties except those who try to work it.

The patients are extraordinarily good, and take everything as it comes (or as it doesn't come!) without any grumbling. Your day is taken up in rapidly deciding which of all the things that want doing you must let go undone; shall they be washed or fed, or beds made, or have their hypodermics and brandies and medicines, or their dressings done? You end in doing some of each in each carriage, or in washing them after dinner instead of before breakfast.

The guns have been banging all the afternoon; some have dropped pretty near again to-day, but you haven't time to take much notice. Our meals are very funny – always candles stuck in a wine bottle – no tablecloth – everything on one plate with the same knife and fork – coffee in a glass, served by a charming dirty Frenchman; many jokes going on between the three tables – the French officials, the M.O.'s, and us. Our own bunks are quite civilised and cosy, though as small as half a big bathing-machine – swept out by our batman.

We have some French wounded and sick on the train.

I see some parsons are enlisting in the R.A.M.C. I hope they know how to scrub floors, clean lavatories, dish out the meals, sleep on the floor, go without baths, live on Maconochie rations, and heave bales and boxes about, and carry stretchers; the orderlies have a very hard life – and no glory.

Must turn in.

Sunday, October 18th, 9 p.m.
Got under way at 6 a.m., and are now about half-way between Paris and Rouen. We outskirted Paris. Passed a train full of Indian troops. Put off the four wounded women at Paris; they have been a great addition to the work, but very sweet and brave; the orderlies couldn't do enough for them; they adored them, and were so indignant at their being wounded. Another man died to-day – shot through the pelvis. One of the enterics, a Skye man, thinks I'm his mother; told me to-night there was a German spy in his carriage, and that he had '50 dead Jocks to bury – and it wasn't the buryin' he didn't like but the feeling of it'. He babbles continually of Germans, ammunition, guns, Jocks, and rations.

Sunday is not Sunday, of course, on a train: no Padre, no services, no nothing – not even any Time. The only thing to mark it to-day is one of the Civil Surgeons wearing his new boots.

We shan't get any letters yet till we get to the new railhead. I'm hoping we shall get time at Rouen to see the Cathedral, do some shopping, have a bath and a shampoo, but probably shan't.

Monday, October 19th.
Rouen, 9 p.m. Got here late last night, and all the wounded were taken off straight away to the two general hospitals here.

One has 1300 cases, and has kept two people operating day

and night. A great many deaths from tetanus.

Seen General French's 2nd despatch (of September) to-day in *Daily Mail*. No mail in, alas! Had a regular debauch in cathedrals and baths to-day. This is the most glorious old city, two cathedrals of surpassing beauty, lovely old streets, broad river, hills, and lovely hot baths and hair shampooing. What with two cathedrals, a happy hour in a hot bath, a shampoo, and delicious tea in the town, we've had a happy day. The train stays here to-night and we are off to-morrow? for ——?

On No.— Ambulance Train (2)

First Battle of Ypres

October 20, 1914, to November 17, 1914

Rouen—First Battle of Ypres—At Ypres—A rest—A General Hospital.

Tuesday, October 20th, 6 p.m.
Just leaving Rouen for Boulogne. We've seen some of the Indians. The Canadians seem to be still on Salisbury Plain. No one knows what we're going to Boulogne empty for.

We have been busy to-day getting the train ready, stocking dressings, &c. All the 500 blankets are sent in to be fumigated after each journey, and 500 others drawn instead. And well they may be; one of the difficulties is the lively condition of the men's shirts and trousers (with worse than fleas) when they come from the trenches in the same clothes they've worn for five weeks or more. You can't wonder we made tracks for a bath at Rouen.

We've just taken on two Belgian officers who want a lift to Boulogne.

Wednesday, October 21st.
Arrived at Boulogne 6 a.m. Went on to Calais, and reached St Omer at 2 p.m., where I believe we are to take up from the motor ambulances. A train of Indians is here. Some Belgian refugees boarded the train at Boulogne, and wanted a lift to

Calais, but had to be turned off reluctantly on both sides. Have been going through bedding equipment to-day.

No mail for me yet, but the others have had one to-day.

3.30 p.m. Off for Steenwerck, close to the Belgian frontier, N.W. of Lille. Good business. Just seen five aeroplanes. Have been warned by Major —— to wear brassards in prominent place, owing to dangerous journey in view!

4.30. This feels like the Front again. Thousands and thousands of Indian troops are marching close to the line, with long fair British officers in turbans, mounted, who salute us, and we wave back; transport on mules. Gorgeous sunset going on; perfectly flat country; no railway traffic except *de la Guerre*.

6 p.m., *Steenwerck*. Pitch dark; saw big guns flashing some way off. The motor ambulances are not yet in with the wounded. The line is cut farther on.

8 p.m. We have had dinner, and have just been down the line to see the place about 100 yards off. The Germans were here six days ago; got into a big sewer that goes under the line, and blew it up. There is a hole 30 feet long, 15 across and 15 deep – very good piece of work. They occupied the station, and bragged about getting across to England from Calais. The M.O. who lives here, to be the link (with a sergeant and seven men) between the field ambulances and the trains, dined with us. It is a wee place. The station is his headquarters.

Thursday, October 22nd.

Took on from convoys all night in pitch darkness – a very bad load this time; going to go septic; swelling under the bandages. There was a fractured spine and a malignant œdema, both dying; we put these two off to-day at St Omer. We came straight away in the morning, and are now nearly back at Boulogne.

YPRES.

Friday, October 23rd.

All unloaded by 11 p.m. last night. (1800 in a day and a night.)

No.— A.T. was in; visited M. and S. Bed by 12; clothes on for forty hours. Slept alongside quay. Two hospital ships in; watched them loading up from ambulances. No time to go ashore. The wounded officers we had this time said the fighting at the Front is very heavy. The men said the same. They slept from sheer exhaustion almost before their boots were got off, and before the cocoa came round. In the morning they perked up very pleased with their sleep, and talked incessantly of the trenches, and the charges, and the odds each regiment had against them, and how many were left out of their company, and all the most gruesome details you can imagine. They seem to get their blood up against the Germans when they're actually doing the fighting – 'You're too excited to notice what hits you, or to think of anything but your life.' ('And your country,' one man added.) 'Some of us has got to get killed, and some wounded, and some captured, and we wonder which is for us.'

11.15. Just off for ——? I was in the act of trotting off into the town to find the baths, when I met a London Scottish with a very urgent note for the O.C.; thought I'd better bide a wee, and it was to say 'Your train is urgently required; how soon can you start?' So I had a lucky escape of being left behind. (We had leave till 1 p.m.) Then the Major nearly got left; we couldn't start that minute, because our stores weren't all in, and the R.T.O. came up in a great fuss that we were holding up five supply trains and reinforcements; so the British Army had to wait for us.

The worst discomforts of this life are (*a*) cold; (*b*) want of drinking water when you're thirsty; (*c*) the appalling atmosphere of the French dining-car; (*d*) lack of room for a bath, and difficulty of getting hot water; (*e*) dirt; (*f*) eccentricities in the meals; (*g*) bad (or no) lights; (*h*) difficulties of getting laundry done; (*i*) personal capture of various live stock; (*j*) broken nights; (*k*) want of exercise on the up journey. Against all these minor details put being at the Front, and all that that includes of thrilling interest – being part of the machinery to give the men the first care and comparative comfort since they landed, at the time they most need it – and least expect it.

6 p.m. Hazebrouck again. We are said to be going to Belgium this time – possibly Ypres. There are a terrible lot of wounded to be got down – more than all the trains can take; they are putting some of them off on the stations where there is a M.O. with a few men, and going back for more.

There were two lovely French torpedo-boats alongside of us at Boulogne.

7.30 p.m., Ypres. Just arrived, all very bucked at being in Belgium. An armoured train, protective coloured all over in huge dabs of red, blue, yellow, and green against aeroplanes, is alongside of us in the station, manned by thirty men R.N.; three trucks are called Nelson, Jellicoe, and Drake, with guns. They look fine; the men say it is a great game. They are directed where to fire at German positions or batteries, and as soon as they answer, the train nips out of range. They were very jolly, and showed us their tame rabbit on active service. They have had no casualties so far. Our load hasn't come in yet. We are *two miles* from our fighting line. No firing to-night to be heard – soon began, though.

Sunday, October 25th.

Couldn't write last night: the only thing was to try and forget it all. It has been an absolute hell of a journey – there is no other word for it. First, you must understand that this big battle from Ostend to Lille is perhaps the most desperate of all, though that is said of each in turn – Mons, the Aisne, and this; but the men and officers who have been through all say this is the worst. The Germans are desperate, and stick at nothing, and the Allies are the same; and in determination to drive them back, each man personally seems to be the same. Consequently the 'carnage' is being appalling, and we have been practically in it, as far as horrors go. Guns were cracking and splitting all night, lighting up the sky in flashes, and fires were burning on both sides. The Clearing Hospital close by, which was receiving the wounded from the field and sending them on to us, was packed and overflowing with badly wounded, the M.O. on the station said.

We had 368; a good 200 were dangerously and seriously wounded, perhaps more; and the sitting-up cases were bad enough. The compound-fractured femurs were put up with rifles and pick-handles for splints, padded with bits of kilts and straw; nearly all the men had more than one wound – some had ten; one man with a huge compound fracture above the elbow had tied on a bit of string with a bullet in it as a tourniquet above the wound himself. When I cut off his soaked three layers of sleeve there was no dressing on it at all.

They were bleeding faster than we could cope with it; and the agony of getting them off the stretchers on to the top bunks is a thing to forget. We were full up by about 2 a.m., and then were delayed by a collision up the line, which was blocked by dead horses as a result. All night and without a break till we got back to Boulogne at 4 p.m. next day (yesterday) we grappled with them, and some were not dressed when we got into B——. The head cases were delirious, and trying to get out of the window, and we were giving strychnine and morphia all round. Two were put off dying at St Omer, but we kept the rest alive to Boulogne. The outstanding shining thing that hit you in the eye all through was the universal silent pluck of the men; they stuck it all without a whine or complaint or even a comment: it was, 'Would you mind moving my leg when you get time,' and 'Thank you very much,' or 'That's absolutely glorious,' as one boy said on having his bootlace cut, or 'That's grand,' when you struck a lucky position for a wound in the back. One badly smashed up said contentedly, 'I was lucky – I was the only man left alive in our trench'; so was another in another trench; sixteen out of twenty-five of one Company in a trench were on the train, all seriously wounded except one. One man with both legs smashed and other wounds was asked if it was all by one shell: 'Oh yes; why, the man next me was blowed to bits.' The bleeding made them all frightfully thirsty (they had only been hit a few hours many of them), and luckily we had got in a good supply of boiled water beforehand on each carriage, so we had plenty when there was time to get it. In the middle of the worst of it in the night I became conscious of a Belgian Boy Scout of fourteen in the corridor, with a glass and a pail of drinking water; that boy worked for hours with his glass and pail on his own, or wherever you sent him. We took him back to Calais. He had come up into the firing line on his cycle fitted with a rifle, with tobacco for the troops, and lived with the British whom he loved, sharing their rations. He was a little brick; one of the Civil Surgeons got him taken back with us, where he wanted to go.

There were twenty-five officers on the train. They said there were 11,000 Germans dead, and they were using the dead piled up instead of trenches.

About 1 o'clock that night we heard a rifle shot: it was a German spy shooting at the sentry sailor on the armoured train alongside of us; they didn't catch him.

It took from 4 to 10 p.m. to unload our bad cases and get them into hospitals on motor ambulances: they lay in rows on their stretchers on the platform waiting their turn without a grumble.

There have been so many hundreds brought down this week that they've had suddenly to clear four hotels for hospitals.

We are now in the filthiest of sidings, and the smell of the burning of our heaps of filthy *débris* off the train is enough to make you sick. We all slept like logs last night, and could have gone on all day; but the train has to be cleaned down by the orderlies, and everything got ready for the next lot: they nearly moved us up again last night, but we shall go to-day.

I think if one knew beforehand what all this was going to be like one would hardly want to face it, but somehow you're glad to be there.

We were tackling a bad wound in the head, and when it was finished and the man was being got comfortable, he flinched and remarked, 'That leg is a beast.' We found a compound-fractured femur put up with a rifle for a splint! He had blankets on, and had never mentioned that his thigh was broken. It too had to be packed, and all he said was, 'That leg *is* a beast,' and, 'That leg is a *Beast*.'

Monday, the 26th, 7 a.m., Ypres. We got here again about 10 p.m. last night in pouring wet, and expected another night like Friday night, but we for some reason remained short of the station, and when we found there was nothing doing, lay down in our clothes and slept, booted and spurred in mackintosh, aprons, &c. We were all so tired and done up yesterday, M.O.'s, Sisters, and orderlies, that we were glad of the respite. There was a tremendous banging and flashing to the north about three o'clock, and this morning it was very noisy, and shaking the train. Some of it sounds quite close. It is a noise you rather miss when it leaves off.

One of the last lot of officers told us he had himself seen in a barn three women and some children, all dead, and all with no hands.

The noise this morning is like a continuous roll of thunder interrupted by loud bangs, and the popping of the French *mitrailleuses*, like our Maxims. The nearest Tommy can get to that word is 'mileytrawsers'. There are two other A.T.'s in, but I hear we are to load up first.

This place is full of Belgian women and children refugees in a bad way from exhaustion.

A long line of our horse ambulances is coming slowly in.

Had a very interesting morning. Got leave to go into the town and see the Cathedral of St Martin. None of the others would budge from the train, so I went alone; town chock-full of French and Belgian troops, and unending streams of columns, also Belgian refugees, cars full of staff officers. The Cathedral is thirteenth century, glorious as usual. There are hundreds of German prisoners in the town in the Cloth Hall. It was a very warrish feeling saying one's prayers in the Cathedral to the sound of the guns of one of the greatest battles in the world.

An M.O. from the Clearing Hospital, with a haggard face, asked me if I could give him some eau-de-Cologne and Bovril for a wounded officer with a gangrenous leg – lying on the station. Sister X. and I took some down, also morphia, and fed them all – frightful cases on stretchers in the waiting-room. They are for our train when we can get in. He told me he had never seen such awful wounds, or such numbers of them. They are being brought down in carts or anything. He said there are 1500 dead Germans piled up in a field five miles off. They say that German officers of ten days' service are commanding.

Tuesday, October 27th, Boulogne.
We got loaded up and off by about 7 p.m., and arrived back here this morning. There are two trains to unload ahead of us, so we shall probably be on duty all day. It is the second night running we haven't had our clothes off – though we did lie down the night before. Last night we had each a four-hour shift to lie down, when all the worst were seen to. One man died at 6 a.m. and another is dying: many as usual are delirious, and the hæmorrhage was worse than ever: it is frightfully difficult to stop it with these bad wounds and compound fractures. One sergeant has both eyes gone from a shell wound.

The twelve sitting-up cases on each carriage are a joy after the tragedy of the rest. They sit up talking and smoking till late, 'because they are so surprised and pleased to be alive, and it is too comfortable to sleep!'

One man with a broken leg gave me both his pillows for a worse man, and said, 'I'm not bad at all – only got me leg broke.' A Reading man, with his face wounded and one eye gone, kept up a running fire of wit and hilarity during his dressing about having himself photographed as a Guy Fawkes for 'Sketchy Bits'.

Wednesday, October 28th.
Got to Boulogne yesterday morning; then followed a most difficult day. It was not till 10 p.m. that they began to unload the sick. The unloading staff at Boulogne have been so overworked night and day that trains get piled up waiting to be unloaded. Fifty motor ambulances have been sent for to the Front, and here they have to depend largely on volunteer people with private motors. Then trains get blocked by other trains each side of them, and nothing short of the fear of death will move a French engine-driver to do what you want him to do. Meanwhile two

men on our train died, and several others were getting on with it, and all the serious cases were in great distress and misery. As a crowning help the train was divided into three parts, each five minutes' walk from any other – dispensary on one bit, kitchen on another. Everybody got very desperate, and at last, after superhuman efforts, the train was cleared by midnight, and we went thankfully but wearily to our beds, which we had not got into for the two previous nights.

To-day was fine and sunny, and while the train was getting in stores we went into the town to find a *blanchisserie*, and bought a cake and a petticoat and had a breath of different air. We expect to move up again any time now. Most welcome mails in.

News of De Wet's rebellion to-day. I wonder if Botha will be able to hold it?

The Times of yesterday (which you can get here) and to-day's *Daily Mail* say the fighting beyond Ypres is 'severe', but that gives the British public no glimmering of what it really is. The —— Regiment had three men left out of one company. The men say General —— cried on seeing the remains of the regiments who answered the rolls. And yet we still drive the Germans back.

There is a train full of slightly wounded Indians in: they are cooking chupatties on nothing along the quay. The boats were packed with refugee families yesterday. We had some badly wounded Germans on our train and some French officers. The British Army doesn't intend the Germans to get to Calais, and they won't get.

Thursday, October 29th, Nieppe.
Woke up to the familiar bangs and rattles again – this time at a wee place about four miles from Armentières. We are to take up 150 here and go back to Bailleul for 150 there. It is a lovely sunny morning, but very cold; the peasants are working in the fields as peacefully as at home. An R.A.M.C. lieutenant was killed by a shell three miles from here three days ago. We've just been giving out scarves and socks to some Field Ambulance men along the line.

Just seen a British aeroplane send off a signal to our batteries – a long smoky snake in the sky; also a very big British aeroplane with a machine-gun on her. A German aeroplane dropped a bomb into this field on Tuesday, meant for the Air Station here. This is the Headquarters of the 4th Division.

Friday, October 30th, Boulogne.
While we were at Nieppe, after passing Bailleul, a German aeroplane dropped a bomb on to Bailleul. After filling up at Nieppe we went back to Bailleul and took up 238 Indians, mostly with smashed left arms from a machine-gun that caught them in the act of firing over a trench. They are nearly all 47th Sikhs, perfect lambs: they hold up their wounded hands and arms like babies for you to see, and insist on having them dressed whether they've just been done or not. They behave like gentlemen, and salaam after you've dressed them. They have masses of long, fine, dark hair under their turbans done up with yellow combs, glorious teeth, and melting dark eyes. One died. The younger boys have beautiful classic Italian faces, and the rest have fierce black beards curling over their ears.

We carried 387 cases this time.

Later. We got unloaded much more quickly to-day, and have been able to have a good rest this afternoon, as I went to bed at 3 a.m. and was up again by 8. It was not so heavy this time, as the Indians were mostly sitting-up cases. Those of a different caste had to sleep on the floor of the corridors, as the others wouldn't have them in. One compartment of four lying-down ones got restless with the pain of their arms, and I found them all sitting up rocking their arms and wailing 'Aie, Aie, Aie,' poor pets. They all had morphia, and subsided. One British Tommy said to me: 'Don't take no notice o' the dirt on me flesh, Sister; I ain't 'ad much time to wash!' quite seriously.

Another bad one needed dressing. I said, 'I won't hurt you.' And he said in a hopeless sort of voice, 'I don't care if you do.' He had been through a little too much.

It is fine getting the same day's London *Daily Mail* here by the Folkestone boat.

It is interesting to hear the individual men express their conviction that the British will never let the Germans through to Calais. They seem as keen as the Generals or the Government. That is why we have had such thousands of wounded in Boulogne in this one week. It is quite difficult to nurse the Germans, and impossible to love your enemies. We always have some on the train. One man of the D.L.I. was bayoneted in three different places, after being badly wounded in the arm by a dumdum bullet. (They make a small entrance hole and burst the limb open in exit.) The man who bayoneted him died in the next bed to him in the Clearing Hospital yesterday morning. You feel that they have all been doing that and worse. We hear at first hand from officers and men specified local instances of unprintable wickedness.

Saturday, October 31st.
Left Boulogne at twelve, and have just reached Bailleul, 6 p.m., where we are to take up wounded Indians again. Somehow they are not so harrowing as the wounded British, perhaps because of the block in language and the weirdness of them. Big guns are booming again. (This was the most critical day of the first battle of Ypres.)

H. sent me a lovely parcel of fifty packets of cigarettes and some chocolate, and A. sent a box of nutmilk choc. They will be grand for the men.

One drawback on having the Indians is that you find them squatting in the corridor, comparing notes on what varieties they find in their clothing! Considering the way one gets smothered with their blankets in the bunks it is the most personally alarming element in the War so far.

Sunday, November 1st, Boulogne – All Saints' Day.
We loaded up with British after all, late in the evening, and had a very heavy night: one of mine died suddenly of femoral hæmorrhage, after sitting up and enjoying his breakfast.

12 noon. We are still unloaded, but I was up all night, and so went out for a blow after breakfast. Found two British T.B.D.'s in dock; on one they were having divine service, close to the quay.

I listened specially to the part about loving our enemies! Then I found the English Church (Colonial and Continental), quite nice and good chants, but I was too sleepy to stay longer than the Psalms: it is ages since one had a chance to go to Church.

After lunch, now they are all unloaded, one will be able to get a stuffy station sleep, regardless of noise and smells.

We carried thirty-nine officers on the train, mostly cavalry, very brave and angelic and polite in their uncomfortable and unwonted helplessness. They liked everything enthusiastically – the beds and the food and the bandages. One worn-out one murmured as he was tucked up, 'By Jove, it is splendid to be out of the sound of those beastly guns; it's priceless.' I had a very interesting conversation with a Major this morning, who was hit yesterday. He says it's only a question of where and when you get it, sooner or later; practically no one escapes.

Rifle firing counts for nothing; it is all the Coal-boxes and Jack Johnsons. The shortage of officers is getting very serious on both sides, and it becomes more and more a question of who can wear out the other in the time.

He said that Aircraft has altered everything in War. German aeroplanes come along, give a little dip over our positions, and away go the German guns. And these innocent would-be peasants working in the fields give all sorts of signals by whirling windmills round suddenly when certain regiments come into action.

The poor L. Regiment were badly cut up in this way yesterday half an hour after coming into their first action; we had them on the train.

They say the French fight well with us, better than alone, and the Indians can't be kept in their trenches; it is up and at 'em. But we shall soon have lost all the men we have out here. Trains and trains full come in every day and night. We are waiting now for five trains to unload. It is a dazzling morning.

Monday, November 2nd.
On way up to ——. The pressure on the Medical Service is now enormous. One train came down to-day (without Sisters) with

1200 sitting-up cases; they stayed for hours in the siding near us without water, cigarettes, or newspapers. You will see in to-day's *Times* that the Germans have got back round Ypres again (where I went into the Cathedral last Monday). No.— A.T. was badly shelled there yesterday. The Germans were trying for the armoured train. The naval officer on the armoured train had to stand behind the engine-driver with a revolver to make him go where he was wanted to. The sitting-up cases on No.— got out and fled three miles down the line. A Black Maria shell burst close to and killed a man. They are again 'urgently needing' A.T.'s; so I hope we are going there to-night.

Eighty thousand German reinforcements are said to have come up to break through our line, and the British dead are now piled up on the field. But they aren't letting the Germans through. Three of our men died before we unloaded at 8 p.m. yesterday, two of shock from lying ten hours in the trench, not dressed.

Tuesday, November 3rd, Bailleul, 8.30 a.m.
Just going to load up; wish we'd gone to Ypres. Germans said to be advancing.

Wednesday, November 4th, Boulogne.
We had a lot of badly wounded Germans who had evidently been left many days; their condition was appalling; two died (one of tetanus), and one British. We have had a lot of the London Scottish, wounded in their first action.

Reinforcements, French guns, British cavalry, are being hurried up the line; they all look splendid.

Wednesday, November 11th.
Sometimes it seems as if we shall never get home, the future is so unwritten.

A frightful explosion like this Hell of a War, which flared up in a few days, will take so much longer to wipe up what can be wiped up. I think the British men who have seen the desolation and the atrocities in Belgium have all personally

settled that it shan't happen in England, and that is why the
headlines always read

'THE BRITISH ARMY IMMOVABLE.'
'WAVES OF GERMAN INFANTRY BROKEN.'
'ALLIES THROW ENEMY BACK AT ALL POINTS.'
'YPRES HELD FOR THREE WEEKS UNDER A RAIN OF
SHELLS.'

You can tell they feel like that from their entire lack of resentment
about their own injuries. Their conversation to each other from
the time they are landed on the train until they are taken off is
never about their own wounds and feelings, but exclusively about
the fighting they have just left. If one only had time to listen or
take it down it would be something worth reading, because it is
not letters home or newspaper stuff, *but told to each other*, with
their own curious comments and phraseology, and no hint of a
gallery or a Press. Incidentally one gets a few eye-openers into
what happens to a group of men when a Jack Johnson lands
a shell in the middle of them. Nearly every man on the train,
especially the badly smashed-up ones, tells you how exceptionally
lucky he was because he didn't get killed like his mate.

Boulogne, Thursday, November 12th, 8 p.m.
Have been here all day. Had a hot bath on the St Andrew.
News from the Front handed down the line coincides with
the *Daily Mail*.

Friday, 13th.
Still here – fourth day of rest. No one knows why; nearly
all the trains are here. The news to-day is glorious. They
say that the Germans did get through into Ypres and were
bayoneted out again.

Friday, November 13th, Boulogne.
We have been all day in Park Lane Siding among the trains,
in pouring wet and slush. I amused myself with a pot of white

paint and a forceps and wool for a brush, painting the numbers on both ends of the coaches inside, all down the train; you can't see the chalk marks at night.

This unprecedented four days' rest and nights in bed is doing us all a power of good; we have books and mending and various occupations.

Saturday, November 14th.
Glorious sunny day, but very cold. Still in Boulogne, but out of Park Lane Siding slum, and among the ships again. Some French sailors off the T.B.'s are drilling on one side of us.

Everything R.A.M.C. at the base is having a rest this week – ships, hospitals, and trains. Major S. said there was not so much doing at the Front – thank Heaven; and the line is still wanted for troops. We have just heard that there are several trains to go up before our turn comes, and that we are to wait about six miles off. Better than the siding anyhow. Meanwhile we can't go off, because we don't know when the train will move out.

The tobacco and the cigarettes from Harrod's have come in separate parcels, so the next will be the chocolate and hankies and cards, &c. It is a grand lot, and I am longing to get up to the Front and give them out.

Sunday, November 15th.
We got a move on in the middle of the night, and are now on our way up.

The cold of this train life is going to be rather a problem. Our quarters are not heated, but we have 'made' (i.e. acquired, looted) a very small oil-stove which faintly warms the corridor, but you can imagine how no amount of coats or clothes keeps you warm in a railway carriage in winter. I'm going to make a foot muff out of a brown blanket, which will help. A smart walk out of doors would do it, but that you can't get off when the train is stationary for fear of its vanishing, and for obvious reasons when it is moving. I did walk round the train for an hour in the dark and slime in the siding yesterday evening, but it is not a cheering form of exercise.

To-day it is *pouring* cats and dogs, awful for loading sick, and there will be many after this week for the trains.

Everyone has of course cleared out of beautiful Ypres, but we are going to load up at Poperinghe, the town next before it, which is now Railhead. Lately the trains have not been so far.

Monday, November 16th, Boulogne, 9 a.m.
We loaded up at Bailleul 344. The Clearing Hospitals were very full, and some came off a convoy. One of mine died. One, wounded above the knee, was four *days* in the open before being picked up; he had six bullets in his leg, two in each arm, and crawled about till found; one of the arm wounds he got doing this. I went to bed at 4. The news was all good, taken as a whole, but the men say they were 'a bit short-handed!' One said gloomily, 'This isn't War, it's Murder; you go there to your doom.' Heard the sad news of Lord Roberts.

We are all the better for our week's rest.

Tuesday, November 17th, 3 a.m.
When we got our load down to Boulogne yesterday morning all the hospitals were full, and the weather was too rough for the ships to come in and clear them, so we were ordered on to Havre, a very long journey. A German died before we got to Abbeville, where we put off two more very bad ones; and at Amiens we put off four more, who wouldn't have reached Havre. About midnight something broke on the train, and we were hung up for hours, and haven't yet got to Rouen, so we shall have them on the train all to-morrow too, and have all the dressings to do for the third time. One of the night orderlies has been run in for being asleep on duty. He climbed into a top bunk (where a Frenchman was taken off at Amiens), and deliberately covered up and went to sleep. He was in charge of 28 patients. Another was left behind at Boulogne, absent without leave, thinking we should unload, and the train went off for Havre. He'll be run in too. Shows how you can't leave the train. Just got to St Just. That looks as if we were going to empty at Versailles instead of Havre.

Lovely starlight night, but very cold. Everybody feels pleased and honoured that Lord Roberts managed to die with us on Active Service at Headquarters, and who would choose a better ending to such a life?

7 a.m. After all, we must be crawling round to Rouen for Havre; passed Beauvais. Lovely sunrise over winter woods and frosted country. Our load is a heavy and anxious one – 344; we shall be glad to land them safely somewhere. The amputations, fractures, and lung cases stand these long journeys very badly.

On No.— Ambulance Train (3)

BRITISH AND INDIANS

November 18, 1914, to December 17, 1914

The Boulogne siding—St Omer—Indian soldiers—His
Majesty King George—Lancashire men on the War—
Hazebrouck—Bailleul—French engine-drivers—Sheepskin
coats—A village in N.E. France—Headquarters.

Wednesday, November 18th, 2 p.m.
At last reached beautiful Rouen, through St Just, Beauvais, and
up to Sergueux, and down to Rouen. From Sergueux through
Rouen to Havre is supposed to be the most beautiful train
journey in France, which is saying a good deal. Put off some
more bad cases here; a boy sergeant, aged 24, may save his
eye and general blood-poisoning if he gets irrigated quickly.
You can watch them going wrong, with two days and two
nights on the train, and it seems such hard luck. And then if
you don't write Urgent or Immediate on their bandages in blue
pencil, they get overlooked in the rush into hospital when they
are landed. So funny to be going back to old Havre, that hot
torrid nightmare of Waiting-for-Orders in August. But, thank
Heaven, we don't stop there, but back to the guns again.

    5 p.m. We are getting on for Havre at last. This long
journey from Belgium down to Havre has been a strange
mixture. Glorious country with the flame and blue haze of

late autumn on hills, towns, and valleys, bare beech-woods with hot red carpets. Glorious British Army lying broken in the train – sleep (or the chance of it) three hours one night and four the next, with all the hours between (except meals) hard work putting the British Army together again; haven't taken off my puttees since Sunday. Seems funny, 400 people (of whom four are women and about sixty are sound) all whirling through France by special train. Why? Because of the Swelled Head of the All-Highest.

We had a boy with no wound, suffering from shock from shell bursts. When he came round, if you asked him his name he would look fixedly at you and say 'yes'. If you asked him something else, with a great effort he said, 'Mother.'

8 p.m. Got to Havre.

Wednesday, 18th November, 6 p.m.
Sotteville, near Rouen. This afternoon's up-journey between Havre and Rouen has been a stripe of pure bliss with no war about it at all. A brilliant dazzling day (which our Island couldn't do if it tried in November), rugs, coat, and cushion on your bed, and the most heavenly view unrolling itself before you without lifting your head to see it, ending up with the lights of Rouen twinkling in the smoke of the factory chimneys under a flaring red sunset.

We are to stop here for repairs to the train – chauffage, electric light, water supply, and gas all to be done. Then we shall be a very smart train. The electric light and the heating will be the greatest help – a chapel and a bathroom I should like added!

At Havre last night the train ran into the Gare Maritime (where we left in the *Asturias* for St Nazaire early in September), which is immediately under the great place that No.— G.H. bagged for their Hospital in August. I ran up and saw it all. It is absolutely first class. There were our people off the train in lovely beds, in huge wards, with six rows of beds—clean sheets, electric light, hot food, and all the M.O.'s, Sisters, and Nursing Orderlies, in white overalls, hard at work on them – orderlies removing their boots and clothing (where we hadn't done it, we leave as much on as we can now because of the cold). Sisters washing them and settling them in, and with the M.O. doing their dressings, all as busy as bees, only stopping to say to us, 'Aren't they brave?' They said we'd brought them an awfully bad lot, and we said we shed all the worst on the way. They don't realise that by the time they get to the base these men are beyond complaining; each stage is a little less infernal to them than the one they've left; and instead of complaining, they tell you how lovely it is! It made one realise the grimness of our stage in it—the emergencies, the makeshifts, and the little four can do for nearly 400 in a train—with their greatest output. We each had 80 lying-down cases this journey.

We got to bed about 11 and didn't wake till nearly 9, to the sound of the No.— G.H. bugle, 'Come to the Cook-House Door, Boys'.

Thursday, November 19th.
Spent the day in a wilderness of railway lines at Sotteville – sharp frost; walk up and down the lines all morning; horizon bounded by fog. This afternoon raw, wet, snowing, slush outside. If it is so deadly cold on this unheated train, what do they do in the trenches with practically the same equipment they came out with in August? Can't last like that. Makes you feel a pig to have a big coat, and hot meals, and dry feet. I've made a fine foot muff with a brown blanket; it is twelve thicknesses sewn together; have still got only summer underclothing. My winter things have been sent on from Havre, but the parcel has not yet reached me; hope the foot muff will ward off chilblains. Got a *Daily Mail* of yesterday. We heard of the smash-up of the Prussian Guard from the people who did it, and had some of the P.G. on our train. Ypres is said to be full of German wounded who will very likely come to us.

Friday, November 20th, 10 a.m., *Boulogne.*
Deep snow.

Boulogne, Saturday, November 21st.

In the siding all yesterday and to-day. Train to be cut down from 650 tons to 450, so we are reconstructing and putting off waggons. It will reduce our number of patients, but we shall be able to do more for a smaller number, and the train will travel better and not waste time blocking up the stations and being left in sidings in consequence. The cold this week has been absolutely awful. The last train brought almost entirely cases of rheumatism. Their only hope at the Front must be hot meals, and I expect the A.S.C. sees that they get them somehow.

A troop train of a very rough type of Glasgow men, reinforcing the Highlanders, was alongside of us early yesterday morning; each truck had a roaring fire of coke in a pail. They were in roaring spirits; it was icy cold.

My winter things arrived from Havre yesterday, so I am better equipped against the cold. Also, this morning an engine gave us an hour or two's chauffage just at getting-up time, which was a help.

Sunday, November 22nd.

Left B. early this morning and got to Merville about midday. Loaded up and got back to B. in the night. Many wounded Germans and a good lot of our sick, knocked over by the cold. I don't know how any of them stick it. Five bombs were dropped the day before where we were to-day, and an old man was killed. Things are being badly given away by spies, even of other nationalities. Some men were sleeping in a cellar at Ypres to avoid the bombardment, with some refugees. In the night they missed two of them. They were found on the roof signalling to the Germans with flash-lights. In the morning they paid the penalty.

The frost has not broken, and it is still bitterly cold.

Tuesday, November 24th.

Was up all Sunday night; unloaded early at Boulogne. Had a bath on a ship and went to bed. Stayed in siding all day.

Wednesday, November 25th.
Left B. about 9.30.

Last night at dinner our charming debonair French garçon was very drunk, and spilt the soup all over me! There was a great scene in French. The fat fatherly corporal (who has a face and expression exactly like the Florentine people in Ghirlandaio's Nativities, and who has the manners of a French aristocrat on his way to the guillotine) tried to control him, but it ended in a sort of fight, and poor Charles got the sack in the end, and has been sent back to Paris to join his regiment. He was awfully good to us Sisters – used to make us coffee in the night, and fill our hot bottles and give us hot bricks for our feet at meals.

Just going on now to a place we've not been to before, called Chocques.

The French have to-day given us an engine with the Red Cross on it and an extra man to attend to the chauffage, so we have been quite warm and lovely. We ply him at the stations with cigarettes and chocolate, and he now falls over himself in his anxiety to please us.

The officers of the two Divisions which are having a rest have got 100 hours' leave in turns. We all now spend hours mapping out how much we could get at home in 100 hours from Boulogne.

Wednesday, November 25th.
Arrived at 11 p.m. last night at a God-forsaken little place about eight miles from the firing line. Found a very depressed major taking a most gloomy view of life and the war, in charge of Indians. Pitch-dark night, and they were a mile away from the station, so we went to bed at 12 and loaded up at 7.30 this morning, all Indians, mostly badly wounded. They are such pathetic babies, just as inarticulate to us and crying as if it was a crêche. I've done a great trade in Hindustani, picked up at a desperate pace from a Hindu officer to-day! If you write it down you can soon learn it, and I've got all the necessary medical jargon now; you read it off, and then spout it without looking at your note-book. The awkward part is when they answer something you haven't got!

The Germans are using sort of steam-ploughs for cutting trenches.

The frost has broken, thank goodness. The Hindu officer said the cold was more than they bargained for, but they were 'very, very glad to fight for England'. He thought the Germans were putting up a very good show. There have been a great many particularly ghastly wounds from hand-grenades in the trenches. We have made a very good journey down, and expect to unload this evening, as we are just getting into Boulogne at 6.30 p.m.

Thursday, November 26th.
We did a record yesterday. Loaded up with the Indians – full load – bad cases – quite a heavy day; back to B. and unloaded by 9 p.m., and off again at 11.30 p.m. No waiting in the siding this time. Three hospital ships were waiting this side to cross by daylight. They can't cross now by night because of enemy torpedoes. So all the hospitals were full again, and trains were taking their loads on to Rouen and Havre. We should have had to if they hadn't been Indians.

We loaded up to-day at Bailleul, where we have been before – headquarters of 3rd and 4th Divisions. We had some time to wait there before loading up, so went into the town and saw the Cathedral – beautiful old tower, hideously restored inside, but very big and well kept. The town was very interesting. Sentries up the streets every hundred yards or so; the usual square packed with transport, and the usual jostle of Tommies and staff officers and motor-cars and lorries. We saw General French go through.

The Surgeon-General had been there yesterday, and five Sisters are to be sent up to each of the two clearing hospitals there. They should have an exciting time. A bomb was dropped straight on to the hospital two days ago – killed one wounded man, blew both hands off one orderly, and wounded another. The airman was caught, and said he was very sorry he dropped it on the hospital; he meant it for Headquarters. We have a lot of cases of frost-bite on the train. One is as bad as in Scott's Expedition; may have to have his foot amputated. I'd never seen it before. They are nearly all slight medical cases; very few wounded, which makes a very light load from the point of view of work, but we shall have them on the train all night. One of us is doing all the train half the night, and another all the train the other half. The other two go to bed all night. I am one of these, as I have got a bit of a throat and have been sent to bed early. We've never had a light enough load for one to do the whole train before. The men say things are very quiet at the Front just now. Is it the weather or the Russian advance?

Great amusement to-day. Major P. got left behind at Hazebrouck, talking to the R.T.O., but scored off us by catching us up at St Omer on an engine which he collared.

Saturday, November 28th.
Sunny and much milder. We came up in the night last night to St Omer, and have not taken any sick on yet. There seems to be only medical cases about just now, which is a blessed relief to think of. They are inevitable in the winter, here or at home. The Major has gone up to Poperinghe with one carriage to fetch six badly wounded officers and four men who were left there the other day when the French took the place over.

I was just getting cigarettes for an up-going train of field-kitchens and guns out of your parcel when it began to move. The men on each truck stood ready, and caught the packets as eagerly as if they'd been diamonds as I threw them in from my train. It was a great game; only two went on the ground. The 'Surprise,' I suppose, is in the round tin. We are keeping it for a lean day.

6 p.m. We are just coming to Chocques for Indians again, not far from Armentières, so I am looking up my Hindustani conversation again.

On Friday – the day between these two journeys – Sister N. and I got a motor ambulance from the T.O. and whirled off to Wimereux in it. It is a lovely place on the sea, about three miles off, now with every hotel, casino, and school taken up by R.A.M.C. Base Hospitals. It was a lovely blue morning, and I went right out to the last rock on the sands and watched the breakers while Sister N. attended to some business. It was glorious after the everlasting railway carriage atmosphere.

Then we found a very nice old church in the town. It is too wet to load up with the Indians to-night, so we have the night in bed, and take them down to-morrow.

A sergeant of the 10th Hussars told me he was in a house with some supposed Belgian refugees. He noticed that when a little bell near the ceiling rang one of them always dashed upstairs. He put a man upstairs to trace this bell and intercept the Belgian. It was connected with the little trap-door of a pigeon-house. When a pigeon came in with a message, this door rang the bell and they went up and got the message. They didn't reckon on having British in the house. They were shot next morning.

It takes me a month to read a Sevenpenny out here.

Sunday (Advent), November 29th.
On the way down from Chocques. We have got Indians, British, and eight Germans this time. One big, handsome, dignified Mussulman wouldn't eat his biscuit because he was in the same compartment as a Hindu, and the Hindu wouldn't eat his because the Mussulman had handed it to him. The Babu I called in to interpret was very angry with both, and called the M. a fool-man, and explained to us that he was telling them that in England 'don't care Mussulman, don't care Hindu' – only in Hindustan, and that if the Captain Sahib said 'eat', it was 'hukm', and they'd got to. My sympathies were with the beautiful, polite, sad-looking M., who wouldn't budge an inch, and only salaamed when the Babu went for him.

Monday, November 30th, Boulogne.
Yesterday a wounded Tommy on the train told me, 'The Jack Johnsons have all gone.' To-day's French communiqué says, 'The enemy's heavy artillery is little in evidence.' There is a less strained feeling about everywhere – a most blessed lull.

We were late getting our load off the train last night, and some were very bad. One of my Sikhs with pneumonia did not live to reach Boulogne. Another pneumonia was very miserable, and kept saying, 'Hindustan gurrum England tanda.' They all think they are in England. The Gurkhas are supposed by the orderlies to be Japanese. They are exactly like Japs, only brown instead of yellow. The orderlies make great friends with them all. One Hindu was singing 'Bonnie Dundee' to them in a little gentle voice, very much out of tune. Their great disadvantage is that they are alive with 'Jack Johnsons' (not the guns). They take off *all* their underclothes and throw them out of the window, and we have to keep supplying them with pyjamas and shirts. They sit and stand about naked, scratching for dear life. It is fatal for the train, because all the cushioned seats are now infected, and so are we. I love them dearly, but it is a big price to pay.

Tuesday, December 1st.

We are to-day in a beautiful high embankment at Wimereux, three miles from Boulogne, right on the sea, and have been dry-docked there till 3 p.m. (when we have just started for?), while endless trains of men and guns have gone up past us. H.M. King George was in the restaurant car of one of them. We have been out all the morning, down to the grey and rolling sea, and have been celebrating December 1st by sitting on the embankment reading back numbers of *The Times*, and one of the C.S.'s and I have been painting enormous Red Crosses on the train.

Punch comes regularly now and is devoured by our Mess. We are very like the apostles, and share everything from cakes and 'Spheres' to remedies for 'Jack Johnsons'. Bread-and-butter doesn't happen, alas!

6.30 p.m. We've just caught up H.M. King George's train at St Omer, but he is evidently out dining with Sir John French. We are just alongside. He has red and blue curtains lining the bridges to keep his royal khaki shoulders from getting smutty. His chef has a grey beard. He is with Poincaré.

Wednesday, December 2nd.

We got to Chocques very late last night and are loading up this morning, but only a few here; we shall stop at Lillers and take more on. We went for our usual exploring walk through seas of mud. There are more big motor-lorries here than I've seen anywhere. We wandered past a place where Indians were busy

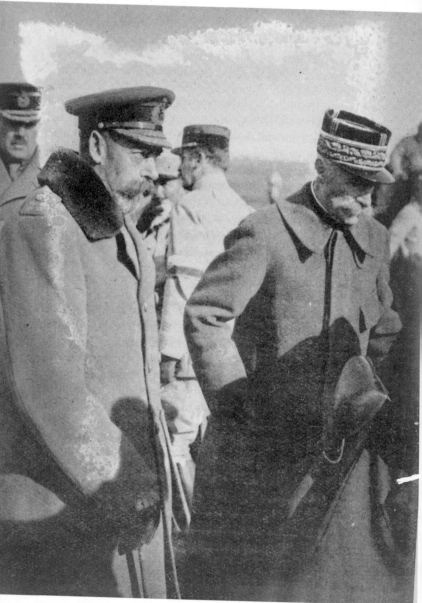

George V visiting troops.

killing and skinning goats – a horrible sight – to one of these châteaux where the staff officers have their headquarters: it was a lovely house in a very clean park; there was a children's swing under the trees and we had some fine swings.

Later. Officers have been on the train on both places begging for newspapers and books. We save up our *Punch*es and *Daily Mail*s and *Times* for them, and give them any Sevenpennies we have to spare. They say at least forty people read each book, and they finish up in the trenches.

H.M. King George was up here yesterday afternoon in a motor and gave three V.C.s.

We have only taken on 83 at the two places. There is so little doing anywhere – no guns have been heard for several days, and there is not much sickness. An officer asked for some mufflers for his Field Ambulance men, so I gave him the rest of the children's: the sailors on the armoured train had the first half. He came back with some pears for us. They are so awfully grateful for the things we give them that they like to bring us something in exchange. Seven men off a passing truck fell over each other getting writing-cases and chocolate to-day. They almost eat the writing-cases with their joy.

9 p.m. We filled up at St Omer from the three hospitals there. A great many cases of frost-bite were put on. They crawl on hands and knees, poor dears. Some left in hospital are very severe and have had to be amputated below the knee. Some of the toes drop off. I have one carriage of twenty-four Indians. A Sikh refused to sit in the same seat with a stout little major of the Gurkhas. I showed him a picture of Bobs, and he said at once, 'Robert Sahib'. They love the *Daily Mirror*s with pictures of Indians. The Sikhs are rather whiney patients and very hard to please, but the little Gurkhas are absolute stoics, and the Bengal Lancers, who are Mohammedans, are splendid.

Thursday, December 3rd.
We kept our load on all night, as we got in very late. I went to bed 10.20 a.m., and then took all the train: unloaded directly after breakfast. Some men from Lancashire were rather interesting on

the war; they thought it would do Europe so much good in the long-run. And the French might try and get their own back when they get into Germany, but 'the British is too tender-'earted to do them things'. They arranged that Belgium should have Berlin! They all get very pitiful over the Belgian homes and desolation; it seems to upset them much more than their own horrors in the trenches. A good deal of the fighting they talk about as if it was an exciting sort of football match, full of sells and tricks and chances. They roar with laughter at some of their escapes.

There was no hospital ship in, which spells a bath or no bath to me, but I ramped round the town till I found a hotel which kindly supplied a fine bath for 1.75. And I found another and nicer English church and a Roman Catholic one.

Grand mail when I came in – from home.

Friday, December 4th.
Had a busy day loading at three places: just going to turn in as I have to be up at 2 a.m.; we shall have the patients on all night. It is a fearful night, pouring and blowing. We have taken a tall white-haired Padre up with us this time: he wanted a trip to the Front. We happened to go to a place we hadn't been to before, in a coal-mining district. While we loaded he marched off to explore, and was very pleased at finding a well-shelled village and an unexploded shell stuck in a tree. It specially seemed to please him to find a church shelled! He has enjoyed talking to the crowds of men on the train on the way down. He lives and messes with us. We opened the Harrod's cake to-day; it is a beauty. The men were awfully pleased with the bull's-eyes, said they hadn't tasted a sweet for four months.

One of the C.S. has just dug me out to see some terrific flashes away over the Channel, which he thinks is a naval battle. I think it is lightning. It was. The gale is terrific: must be giving the ships a doing.

Saturday, December 5th, 7 a.m.
We had a long stop on an embankment in the night, and at last the Chef de Gare from the next station came along the

line and found both the French guards rolled up asleep and the engine-driver therefore hung up. Then he ran out of coal, and couldn't pull the train up the hill, so we had another four hours' wait while another engine was sent for. Got into B. at 6 a.m.; bitterly cold and wet, and no chauffage.

Sunday, December 6th.

A brilliant frosty day – on way up to Bailleul. We unloaded early at B. yesterday, and waited at a good place half-way between B. and Calais, a high down not far from the sea, with a splendid air. Some of the others went for a walk as we had no engine on, but I had been up since 2 a.m., and have hatched another bad cold, and so retired for a sleep till tea-time.

Just got to Hazebrouck. Ten men and three women were killed and twenty wounded here this morning by a bomb. They are very keen on getting a good bag here, especially on the station, and for other reasons, as it is an important junction.

4 p.m. We have been up to B. and there were no patients for us, so we are to go back to the above bomb place to collect theirs. B. was packed with pale, war-worn, dirty but cheerful French troops entraining for their Front. They have been all through everything, and say they want to go on and get it finished. They carry fearful loads, including an extra pair of boots, a whole collection of frying-pans and things, and blankets, picks, &c., all on their backs.

The British officers on the station came and grabbed our yesterday's *Daily Mail*s, and asked for soap, so what you sent came in handy. They went in to the town to buy grapes for us in return. This place is famous for grapes – huge monster purple ones – but the train went out before they came back. We had got some earlier, though.

9 p.m. We are nearly back at Boulogne and haven't taken up any sick or wounded anywhere. One of the trains has taken Indians from Boulogne down to Marseilles – several days' journey.

Monday, December 7th.

Pouring wet day. Still standing by; nothing doing anywhere. It is a blessed relief to know that, and the rest does no one any harm. Had a grand mail to-day.

There is a heart-breaking account of my beautiful Ypres on page 8 of December 1st *Times*. There was a cavalry officer looking round the Cathedral with me that day the guns were banging. I often wonder where the Belgian woman is who showed me the way and wanted my S.A. ribbons as a souvenir. She showed me a huge old painting on the wall of the Cathedral of Ypres in an earlier war.

I all but got left in Boulogne to-day. We are dry-docked about five miles out, not far from Ambleteuse.

It was bad luck not seeing the King. We caught him up at St Omer, and saw his train; and from there he motored in front of us to all our places. Where we went, they said, 'The King was here yesterday and gave V.C.s.' We haven't seen the 'd—d good boy' either.

Tuesday, December 8th.

Got up to Bailleul by 11 a.m., and had a good walk on the line waiting to load up. Glorious morning. Aeroplanes buzzing overhead like bees, and dropping coloured signals about. Only filled up my half of the train, both wounded and sick, including some very bad enterics. An officer in the trenches sent a man on a horse to get some papers from us. Luckily I had a batch of *The Times*, *Spectator*, and *Punches*.

We have come down very quickly, and hope to unload to-night, 9.30.

Wednesday, December 9th.

In siding at Boulogne all day. Pouring wet.

Thursday, December 10th.

Left for Bailleul at 8 a.m. Heard at St Omer of the sinking of the three German cruisers.

Arrived at 2 p.m. Loaded up in the rain, wounded and sick – full load. They were men wounded last night, very muddy and trenchy; said the train was like heaven! It is lovely fun taking the sweets round; they are such an unexpected treat. The sitting-ups make many jokes, and say 'they serve round 'arder sweets than this in the firing line – more explosive like'.

One showed us a fearsome piece of shell which killed his chum next to him last night. There is a good deal of dysentery about, and acute rheumatism. The Clearing Hospitals are getting rather rushed again, and the men say we shall have a lot coming down in the next few days. A hundred men of one regiment got separated from their supports and came up against some German machine-guns in a wood with tragic results. We are shelling from Ypres, but there is no answering shelling going on just now, though the Taubes are busy.

We are wondering what the next railhead will be, and when. Some charming H.A.C.s are on the train this time, and a typically plucky lot of Tommies. One of the best of their many best features is their unfailing friendliness with each other. They never let you miss a man out with sweets or anything if he happens to be asleep or absent.

Friday, December 11th.
They wouldn't unload us at 11 p.m. at Boulogne last night, but sent us on to the Duchess of Westminster's Hospital at a little place about twenty miles south of B., and we didn't unload till this morning. It was my turn for a whole night in bed. Not that this means we are having many nights up, but that when the load doesn't require two Sisters at night, two go to bed and the other two divide the night. After unloading we had a poke round the little fishing village, and of course the church. A company of Canadian Red Cross people unloaded us. The hospital has not been open very long. It was all sand-dunes and fir-trees on the way, very attractive, and cement factories.

Mail in again.

9 p.m. We came back to B. to fill up with stores after lunch, and haven't been sent out again yet; but we often go to bed here, and wake up and ask our soldier servants (batmen), who bring our jugs of hot water it the morning, where we are. I like the motion of the train in bed now, and you get used to the noise.

Saturday, December 12th.

The French engine-drivers are so erratic that if you're long enough on the line it's only a question of time when you get your smash up. Ours came last night when they were joining us up to go out again. They put an engine on to each end of one-half of the train (not the one our car is in), and then did a tug-of-war. That wasn't a success, so they did the concertina touch, and put three coaches out of action, including the kitchen. So we're stuck here now (Boulogne) till Heaven knows when. Fortunately no casualties.

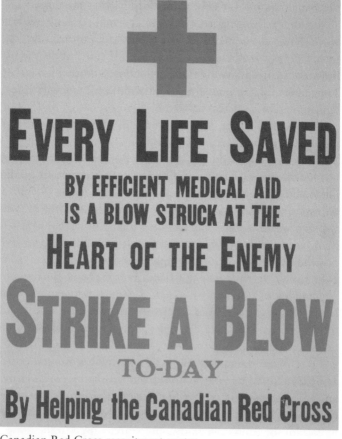

Canadian Red Cross recruitment poster.

Sunday, December 13th.

We've been hung up since Friday night by the three damaged trucks, and took the opportunity of getting some good walks yesterday, and actually going to church at the English church this morning.

Sister B. has been ordered to join the hospital; she mobilised to-day, and we had to pack her off this morning. The staffs of the trains (which have all been shortened) have been put down from four to three. Very glad I wasn't taken off.

We saw a line of graves with wooden crosses, in a field against the skyline, last journey.

We have seen a lot of the skin coats that the men are getting now. Sheepskin, with any sort of fur or skin sleeves, just the skins sewn together; you may see a grey or white coat with brown or black fur or astrakhan sleeves. Some wear the fur inside and some outside; they simply love them.

Reduced to pacing the platform in the dark and rain to get warm. It is 368 paces, so I've done it six times to well cover a mile, but it is not an exciting walk! Funny thing, it seems in this war that for many departments you are either thoroughly overworked or entirely hung up, which is much worse. In things like the Pay Department or the Post-Office or the Provisioning for the A.S.C. it seldom gets off the overworked line, but in this and in the fighting line it varies very much.

> The number of victims of the Taube attack on Hazebrouck on Monday is larger than was at first supposed. Five bombs were thrown and nine British soldiers and five civilians were killed, while 25 persons were injured.
>
> *The Times*, Dec. 9th.

We were at H. on that day.

Monday, December 14th.

Got off at last at 3.30 a.m. Loaded up 300 at Merville, a place we've only been to once before, near the coalmines. Guns were banging only four miles off.

Had a good many bad cases, medical and surgical, this time: kept one busy to the journey's end. We are unloaded to-night, so they will soon be well seen to, instead of going down to Rouen or Havre, which two other trains just in have got to do.

We have a good many Gordons on; one was hugging his bagpipes, and we had him up after dinner to play, which he did beautifully with a wrapt expression.

We are going up again to-night. 'Three trains wanted immediately' – been expecting that.

Tuesday, December 15th.
We were unloaded last night at 9.30, and reported ready to go up again at 11 p.m., but they didn't move us till 5 a.m. Went to same place as yesterday, and cleared the Clearing Hospitals again; some badly wounded, with wounds exposed and splints padded with straw as in the Ypres days.

The Black Watch have got some cherub-faced boys of seventeen out now. The mud and floods are appalling. The Scotch regiments have lost their shoes and spats and wade barefoot in the water-logged trenches. This is a true fact.

I'm afraid not a few of many regiments have got rheumatism – some acute – that they will never lose.

The ploughed fields and roads are all more or less under water, and each day it rains more.

We have got a Red Cross doctor on the train who was in the next village to the one we loaded from this morning. It has been taken and retaken by both sides, and had a population of about 2000. The only living things he saw in it to-day besides a khaki supply column passing through were one cat and some goldfish. In one villa a big brass bedstead was hanging through the drawing-room ceiling by its legs, the clothes hanging in the cupboards were slashed up, and nothing left anywhere. He says at least ten well-to-do men of 50 are doing motor-ambulance work with their own Rolls-Royces up there, and cleaning their cars themselves, at 6 a.m.

I happened to ask a man, who is a stretcher-bearer belonging to the Rifle Brigade, how he got hit. 'Oh, I was carrying a dead man,' he said modestly. 'My officer told me not to move him till dark, because of the sniping; but his face was blown off by an explosive bullet, and I didn't think it would do the chaps who had to stand round him all day any good, so I put him on my back, and they copped me in the leg. I was glad he wasn't a wounded man, because I had to drop him.'

He told me some French ladies were killed in their horse-and-cart on the road near their trenches the other day; they would go and try and get some of their household treasures. Two were killed – two and a man – and the horse wounded. He helped to take them to the R.A.M.C. dressing-station.

Wednesday, December 16th.

We are on our way up again to-day, and by a different and much jollier way, to St Omer, going south of Boulogne and across country, instead of up by Calais. We came back this way with patients from Ypres once. It is longer, but the country is like Hampshire Downs, instead of the everlasting flat swamps the other way. Of course it is raining.

6 p.m. For once we waited long enough at St Omer to go out and explore the beautiful ruined Abbey near the station. We went up the town – very clean compared with the towns farther up – swarming with grey touring-cars and staff officers. Headquarters of every arm labelled on different houses, and a huge church the same date as the Abbey, with some good carving and glass in it. We kept an eye open for Sir J.F. and the P. of W., but didn't meet them. Saw the English military church where Lord Roberts began his funeral service. For once it wasn't raining.

Thursday, December 17th.

Left St O. at 11 p.m. last night, and woke up this morning at Bailleul. Saw two aeroplanes being fired at – black smoke-balls bursting in the air. Heard that Hartlepool and Scarboro' have been shelled – just the bare fact – in last night's *Globe*. R. will have an exciting time. We're longing to get back for to-day's *Daily Mail*.

There has been a lot of fighting in our advance south-east of Ypres since Sunday.

The Gordons made a great bayonet charge, but lost heavily in officers and men in half an hour; we have some on the train. The French also lost heavily, and lie unburied in hundreds; but the men say the Germans were still more badly 'punished'. They tell us that in the base hospitals they never get a clean wound; even the emergency amputations and trephinings and operations done in the Clearing Hospitals are septic, and no one who knew the conditions would wonder at it. We shall all forget what aseptic work is by the time we get home. The anti-tetanus serum injection that every wounded man gets with his first dressing has done a great deal to keep the tetanus under, and the spreading gangrene is less fatal than it was. It is treated with incisions and injections of H_2O_2, or,

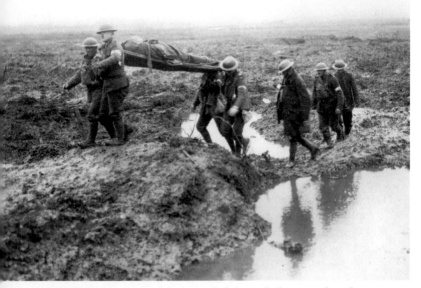

Stretcher bearers carry the wounded through the seas of mud.

when necessary, amputation in case of limbs. You suspect it by the grey colour of the face and by another sense, before you look at the dressing.

At B. a man at the station greeted me, and it was my old theatre orderly at No. 7 Pretoria. We were very pleased to see each other. I fitted him out with a pack of cards, post-cards, acid drops, and a nice grey pair of socks.

A wounded officer told us he was giving out the mail in his trench the night before last, and nearly every man had either a letter or a parcel. Just as he finished a shell came and killed his sergeant and corporal; if they hadn't had their heads out of the trench at that moment for the mail, neither of them would have been hit. The officer could hardly get through the story for the tears in his eyes.

CHRISTMAS AND NEW YEAR ON THE TRAIN

December 18, 1914, to January 3, 1915.

The Army and the King—Mufflers—Christmas Eve—
Christmas on the train—Princess Mary's present—The
trenches in winter—'A typical example'—New Year's Eve at
Rouen—The young officers.

Friday, December 18th, 10.30 a.m.
We've had an all-night journey to Rouen, and have almost
got there. One of my sitting-ups was 106° this morning, but it
was only malaria, first typical one I have met since S.A. A man
who saw the King when he was here said, 'They wouldn't let
him come near the trenches; if a shell had come and hit him I
think the Army would 'a gone mad; there'd be no keeping 'em
in the trenches after that.'

This place before Rouen is Darnetal, a beautiful spiry
town in a valley, pronounced by the Staff of No.— A.T.
'Darn it all'.

6 p.m. We unloaded by 12, and had just had time to go out
and get a bath at the best baths in France.

Shipped a big cargo of J.J. this journey, but luckily made no
personal captures.

Got to sleep this afternoon, as I was on duty all yesterday
and up to 2 a.m.this morning.

Pouring cats and dogs as usual.

No time to see the Cathedrals.

We had this time a good many old seasoned experienced men of the Regular Army, who had been through all the four months (came out in August). They are very strong on the point of mixing Territorials (and K.'s Army where it is not composed of old service men) and Indians well in with men like themselves.

One Company of R.E. lost all its officers in one day in a charge. A H.L.I. man gave a chuckling account of how they got to fighting the Prussian Guard with their fists at Wypers because they were at too close quarters to get in with their bayonets. They really enjoyed it, and the Germans didn't.

Saturday, 19th.

We are dry-docked to-day at Sotteville, outside Rouen. Z. and I half walked and half trammed into Rouen this morning.

It is lovely to get out of the train. This afternoon No.— played a football match against the Khaki train and got well beaten. They've only been in the country six weeks, and only do about one journey every eight days, so they are in better training than ours, but it will do them a lot of good: we looked on.

Sunday, 20th, 6 p.m.

At last we are on our way back to Boulogne and mails, and the News of the War at Home and Abroad. At Rouen, or rather the desert four miles outside it, we only see the paper of the day before, and we miss our mails, and have no work since unloading on Friday. This morning was almost a summer day, warm, still, clear and sunny. We went for a walk, and then got on with painting the red crosses on the train, which can only be done on fine days, of which we've had few. The men were paraded, and then sent route-marching, which they much enjoyed. It was possible, as word was sent that the train was not going out till 1.30. It did, however, move at 12, which shows how little you can depend on it, even when a time is given. They had a mouth-organ and sang all the way.

Monday, December 21st.

Got to Boulogne early this morning after an exceptionally rackety journey, all one's goods and chattels dropping on one's head at intervals during the night. Engine-driver rather *ivré*, I should think. Off again at 10.30 a.m.

Mail in.

Weather appallingly cold and no chauffage.

On way up to Chocques, where we shall take up Indians again. How utterly miserable Indians must be in this eternal wet and cold. The fields and land generally are all half under water again. We missed the last two days' papers, and so have heard nothing of the war at home, except that the casualties are over 60,000. Five mufflers went this afternoon to five men on a little isolated station on the way here. When I said to the first boy, 'Have you got a muffler?' he thought I wanted one for someone on the train.

'Well, it's not a real muffler; it's my sleeping-cap,' he said, beginning to pull it off his neck; 'but you're welcome to it if it's any use!'

What do you think of that? He got pink with pleasure over a real muffler and some cigarettes. You start with two men; when you come back in a minute with the mufflers the two have increased to five silent expectant faces.

Wednesday, 23rd.

We loaded up at Lillers late on Monday night with one of the worst loads we've ever taken, all wounded, half Indians and half British.

You will see by Tuesday's French communiqués that some of our trenches had been lost, and these had been retaken by the H.L.I., Manchesters, and 7th D.G.s.

It was a dark wet night, and the loading people were half-way up to their knees in black mud, and we didn't finish loading till 2 a.m., and were hard at it trying to stop hæmorrhage, &c., till we got them off the train at 11 yesterday morning; the J.J.'s were swarming, but a large khaki pinny tying over my collar, and with elastic wristbands, saved me this time. One little Gurkha with his arm just amputated, and a wounded leg, could only be pacified by having acid drops put into his mouth and being allowed to hug the tin.

Another was sent on as a sitting-up case. Half-way through the night I found him gasping with double pneumonia; it was no joke nursing him with seven others in the compartment. He only just lived to go off the train.

Another one I found dead about 5.30 a.m. We were to have been sent on to Rouen, but the O.C. Train reported too many serious cases, and so they were taken off at B. It was a particularly bad engine-driver too.

I got some bath water from a friendly engine, and went to bed at 12 next day.

We were off again the same evening, and got to B. this morning, train full, but not such bad cases, and are on our way back again now: expect to be sent on to Rouen. Now we are three instead of four Sisters, it makes the night work heavier, but we can manage all right in the day. In the last journey some of the worst cases got put into the top bunks, in the darkness and rush, and one only had candles to do the dressings by. One of the C.S.'s was on leave, but has come back now. All the trains just then had bad loads: the Clearing Hospitals were overflowing.

The Xmas Cards have come, and I'm going to risk keeping them till Friday, in case we have patients on the train. If not, I shall take them to a Sister I know at one of the B. hospitals.

We have got some H.A.C. on this time, who try to stand up when you come in, as if you were coming into their drawing-room. The Tommies in the same carriage are quite embarrassed. One boy said just now, 'We 'ad a 'appy Xmas last year.'

'Where?' I said.

'At 'ome, 'long o' Mother,' he said, beaming.

Xmas Eve, 1914.

And no fire and no chauffage, and cotton frocks; funny life, isn't it? And the men are crouching in a foot of water in the trenches and thinking of "ome, 'long o' Mother,' – British, Germans, French, and Russians. We are just up at Chocques going to load up with Indians again. Had more journeys this week than for a long time; you just get time to get what sleep the engine-driver and the cold will allow you on the way up.

8 p.m. Just nearing Boulogne with another bad load, half Indian, half British; had it in daylight for the most part, thank goodness! Railhead to-day was one station further back than last time, as the —— Headquarters had to be evacuated after the Germans got through on Sunday. The two regiments, Coldstream Guards and Camerons, who drove them back, lost heavily and tell a tragic story. There are two men (only one is a boy) on the train who got wounded on Monday night (both compound fracture of the thigh) and were only taken out of the trench this morning, Thursday, to a Dressing Station and then straight on to our train. (We heard the guns this morning.) Why they are alive I don't know, but I'm afraid they won't live long: they are sunken and grey-faced and just strong enough to say, 'Anyway, I'm out of the trench now.' They had drinks of water now and then in the field but no dressings, and lay in the slush. Stretcher-bearers are shot down immediately, with or without the wounded, by the German snipers.

And this is Christmas, and the world is supposed to be civilised. They came in from the trenches to-day with blue faces and chattering teeth, and it was all one could do to get them warm and fed. By this evening they were most of them revived enough to enjoy Xmas cards; there were such a nice lot that they were able to choose them to send to Mother and My Young Lady and the Missis and the Children, and have one for themselves.

The Indians each had one, and salaamed and said, 'God save you,' and 'I will pray to God for you,' and 'God win your enemies,' and 'God kill many Germans,' and 'The Indian men too cold, kill more Germans if not too cold.' One with a S.A. ribbon spotted mine and said, 'Africa same like you.'

Midnight. Just unloaded, going to turn in; we are to go off again at 5 a.m.to-morrow, so there'll be no going to church. Mail in, but not parcels; there's a big block of parcels down at the base, and we may get them by Easter.

With superhuman self-control I have not opened my mail to-night so as to have it to-morrow morning.

Xmas Day, 11 a.m.

On way up again to Béthune, where we have not been before (about ten miles beyond where we were yesterday), a place I've always hoped to see. Sharp white frost, fog becoming denser as we get nearer Belgium. A howling mob of reinforcements stormed the train for smokes. We threw out every cigarette, pipe, pair of socks, mits, hankies, pencils we had left; it was like feeding chickens, but of course we hadn't nearly enough.

Everyone on the train has had a card from the King and Queen in a special envelope with the Royal Arms in red on it. And this is the message (in writing hand)

With our best wishes for Christmas, 1914.
May God protect you and bring you home safe.
MARY R. GEORGE R.I.

That is something to keep, isn't it?

An officer has just told us that those men haven't had a cigarette since they left S'hampton, hard luck. I wish we'd had enough for them. It is the smokes and the rum ration that has helped the British Army to stick it more than anything, after the conviction that they've each one got that the Germans have got to be 'done in' in the end. A Sergt. of the C.G. told me a cheering thing yesterday. He said he had a draft of young soldiers of only four months' service in this week's business. 'Talk of old soldiers,' he said, 'you'd have thought these had had years of it. When they were ordered to advance there was no stopping them.'

After all we are not going to Béthune but to Merville again.

This is a very slow journey up, with long indefinite stops; we all got bad headaches by lunch time from the intense cold and a short night following a heavy day. At lunch we had hot bricks for our feet, and hot food inside, which improved matters, and I think by the time we get the patients on there will be chauffage.

The orderlies are to have their Xmas dinner to-morrow, but I believe ours is to be to-night, if the patients are settled up in time.

Do not think from these details that we are at all miserable; we say 'For King and Country' at intervals, and have many jokes over it all, and there is the never-failing game of going over what we'll all do and avoid doing After the War.

7 p.m.—Loaded up at Merville and now on the way back; not many badly wounded but a great many minor medicals, crocked up, nothing much to be done for them. We may have to fill up at Hazebrouck, which will interrupt the very festive Xmas dinner the French Staff are getting ready for us. It takes a man, French or British, to take decorating really seriously. The orderlies have done wonders with theirs. Aeroplanes done in cotton-wool on brown blankets is one feature.

This lot of patients had Xmas dinner in their Clearing Hospitals to-day, and the King's Xmas card, and they will get Princess Mary's present. Here they finished up D.'s Xmas cards and had oranges and bananas, and hot chicken broth directly they got in.

12 Midnight. Still on the road. We had a very festive Xmas dinner, going to the wards which were in charge of nursing orderlies between the courses. Soup, turkey, peas, mince pie, plum pudding, chocolate, champagne, absinthe, and coffee. Absinthe is delicious, like squills. We had many toasts in French and English. The King, the President, Absent Friends, Soldiers and Sailors, and I had the *Blessés* and the *Malades*. We got up and clinked glasses with the French Staff at every toast, and finally the little chef came in and sang to us in a very sweet musical tenor. Our great anxiety is to get as many orderlies and N.C.O.s as possible through the day without being run in for drunk, but it is an uphill job; I don't know where they get it.

We are wondering what the chances are of getting to bed to-night.

4 a.m.—Very late getting in to B.; not unloading till morning. Just going to turn in now till breakfast time. End of Xmas Day.

Saturday, December 26th.
Saw my lambs off the train before breakfast. One man in the

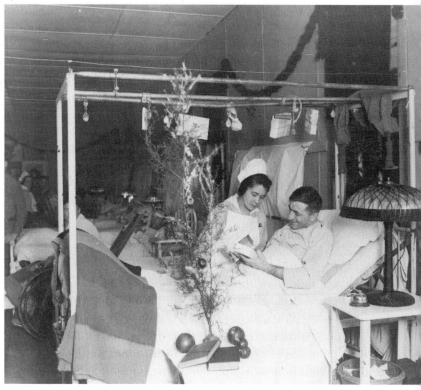

Christmas in hospital.

Warwicks had twelve years' service, a wife and two children, but 'when Kitchener wanted more men' he re-joined. This week he got an explosive bullet through his arm, smashing it up to rags above the elbow. He told me he got a man 'to tie the torn muscles up', and then started to crawl out, dragging his arm behind him. After some hours he came upon one of his own officers wounded, who said, 'Good God, sonny, you'll be bleeding to death if we don't get you out of this; catch hold of me and the Chaplain.' 'So 'e cuddled me, and I cuddled the Chaplain, and we got as far as the doctor.'

At the Clearing H. his arm was taken off through the shoulder-joint, but I'm afraid it is too late. He is now a pallid wreck, dying of gangrene. But he would discuss the War, and when it would end, and ask when he'd be strong enough to sit up and write to that officer, and apologised for wanting drinks so often. He is one of the most top-class gallant gentlemen it's ever been my jolly good luck to meet. And there are hundreds of them.

We had Princess Mary's nice brass box this morning. The V.A.D. here brought a present to every man on the train this morning, and to the orderlies. They had 25,000 to distribute, cigarette-cases, writing-cases, books, pouches, &c. The men were frightfully pleased, it was so unexpected. The processions of hobbling, doubled-up, silent, muddy, sitting-up cases who pour out of the trains want something to cheer them up, as well as the lying-downs. It is hard to believe they are the fighting men, now they've handed their rifles and bandoliers in. (It is snowing fast.) We have to go and drink the men's health at their spread at 1 o'clock. Then I hope a spell of sleep.

We have chauffage on to-day to thaw the froidage; the pipes are frozen.

6 p.m. We all processed to the Orderlies' Mess truck and the O.C. made a speech, and the Q.M.S. dished out drinks for us to toast with, and we had the King and all of ourselves with great enthusiasm. Mr T. had to propose 'The Sisters', and after a few trembling, solemn words about 'we all know the good work they do', he suddenly giggled hopelessly, and it ended in a healthy splodge all round. Orders just come to be at St Omer by 10 p.m. If that means loading-up further on about 1 a.m.I think we shall all die! Too noisy here to sleep this afternoon. And the men are just now so merry with Tipperary, and dressing up, that they will surely drop the patients off the stretchers, but we'll hope for the best.

Sunday, December 27th.
Had a grand night last night. Woke up at Béthune. Went out after breakfast and saw over No.— Cl. H., which has only been there 48 hours, in a huge Girls' College, partly smashed by big shell holes, an awful mess, but the whole parts are being turned into a splendid hospital. Several houses shelled, and big guns

shaking the train this morning.

The M.O.'s went to the Orderlies' Concert last night, when we went to bed. It was excellent, and nobody was drunk! We are taking on a full load of lying-downs straight from three Field Ambulances, so we shall be very busy; not arrived yet.

6 p.m. Nearing Boulogne.

I have one little badly wounded Gurkha (who keeps ejaculating 'Gerrman'), and all the rest British, some very badly frost-bitten. The trenches are in a frightful state. One man said, 'There's almost as many men drowned as killed: when they're wounded they fall into the water.' Of three officers (one of whom is on the train and tells the story) in a deep-water trench for two days, one was drowned, the other had to have his clothes cut off him (stuck fast to the mud) and be pulled out naked, and the other is invalided with rheumatism.

Two men were telling me how they caught a sniper established in a tree, with a thousand rounds of ammunition and provisions. He asked for mercy, but he didn't get it, they said. He had just shot two stretcher-bearers.

Monday, December 28th.
This trip to Rouen will give us a longer journey up, and therefore some more time. And we shall get another bath.

The following story is a typical example of what the infantry often have to endure. It was told to me by the Sergeant. Three men of the S.W. Borderers and five of the Welsh Regt. on advancing to occupy a trench found themselves cut off, with a 2nd Lieut. He advanced alone to reconnoitre and was probably shot, they said – they never saw him again. So the Sergt. of the W.R. (aged 22!) took command and led them for safety, still under fire, to a ditch with one foot of water in it. This was on the *Monday night before Xmas*. They stayed in it all Tuesday and Tuesday night, when it was snowing. Before daylight he 'skirmished' them to a trench he knew of two hundred yards in advance, where he had seen one of his regiment the day before. This was in water above their knees. He showed me the mud-line on his trousers.

This turned out to be one of the German communication trenches. They stayed in that all Wednesday, Wednesday night, and Thursday, living on some biscuit one man had, some bits of chocolate, and drinking the dirty trench water, in which was a dead German dressed as a Gurkha. 'We was prayin' all the time,' said one of them. Then one ventured out to get water and was shot. On Xmas Eve night it froze hard, and they were so weak and starved and numb that the Sergt. decided that they couldn't stick it any longer, so they cast their equipment and made a dash for a camp fire they could see.

One of them is an old grey-haired Reservist with seven children. By good luck they struck a road which led them to some Coldstreams' billet, a house. There they were fed with tea, bread, bacon, and jam, and stayed an hour, but didn't get dried.

Then these C.G.'s had to go into action, and the Sergt. took them on to some Grenadier Guards' billet. By this time he and one other had to be carried by the others. There they stayed the night (Xmas Day) and saw the M.O.'s of a Field Ambulance, who sent them all into hospital at Béthune, whence we took them on this train to Rouen, all severely frost-bitten, weak, and rheumatic.

An infant boy of nineteen was telling me how he killed a German of 6 ft. 3 in. '"Bill," I says, "there's one o' them big devils," ('only I called him worse than that,' he said politely to me), and we all three emptied our rifles into him, and he never moved again.'

9 p.m. At Sotteville, off Rouen. We got unloaded at 1 p.m. and then made a dash for the best baths in France.

Tuesday, December 29th.
We've had a quite useful day off to-day. Still at Sotteville; had a walk this morning, also got through arrears of mending and letter-writing. They played another football match this afternoon, and did much better than last time, but still got beaten.

Wednesday, December 30th.
Still at Sotteville. One of our coaches is off being repaired here,

and goodness knows how long we shall be stuck.

Had a walk this morning along the line. The train puffed past me on its way to Rouen for water. I tried to make the engine-driver stop by spreading myself out in front of the engine, but he 'shooed' me out of the way, and after some deliberation I seized a brass rail and leapt on to the footboard about half-way down the train; it wasn't at all difficult after all. We had Seymour Hicks' lot tacked on behind us; they are doing performances for the Hospitals and Rest-camps in Rouen to-day, but unfortunately we are too far out to go in.

Thursday, December 31st, New Year's Eve.
Still at Sotteville, and clemmed with cold. There was no paraffin on the train this morning, so we couldn't even have the passage lamps lit.

This afternoon I went with Major —— and the French Major and the little fat French Caporal (who is the same class as the French Major—or better) into Rouen, and they trotted us round sight-seeing. The little Caporal showed us all the points of the cathedrals, and the twelfth-century stone pictures on the north porch and on the towers, and also the church of St Maclou with the wonderful 'Ossuare' cloisters, now a college for Jeunes Filles. We had tea in the town and trammed back. This evening, New Year's Eve, the French Staff had decorated the Restaurant with Chinese lanterns, and we had a festive New Year's Eve dinner, with chicken, and Xmas pudding on fire, and Sauterne and Champagne and crackers. The putting on of caps amused every one *infiniment*, and we had more speeches and toasts. I forgot to tell you that the French Major's home is broken up by *les Allemands*, and he doesn't know where his wife and three children are. On Xmas night, during toasts, he suddenly got up and said in a broken voice, 'À mes petits enfants et ma femme.'

The coach is mended and back from *l'atelier*, and we may go off at any moment. I hope we shall wake up on the way to Boulogne and mails.

New Year's Day, 1915, Rouen.
A Happy New Year to us all! We are not off yet, and several other trains are doing nothing here. We came into Rouen this afternoon, and heard that we are to clear the hospitals here to-morrow, and take them down to Havre.

Thank goodness we are to move at last. Went for a walk in the town after tea, and after dinner the O.C. and Sister B. and one of the Civil Surgeons and the French Major and I went to the cinema. It was excellent, or we thought it so, after the months of train and nothing else.

Saturday, January 2nd, 12 noon.
Just loading up for Havre with many of the same men we brought down from Béthune on Sunday; it seems as if we might just as well have taken them straight down to Havre. They look clean now, and have lost the trench look.

Have been asked to say how extra-excellent the Xmas cake was; we finished it yesterday, ditto the Tiptree jam.

It is a week on Monday since we had any mails.

There is a Major of ours on the train, getting a lift to Havre, who is specialist in pathology, and he has been investigating the bacillus of malignant œdema and of spreading gangrene. They are hunting anærobes (Sir Almroth Wright at Boulogne and a big French Professor in Paris) for a vaccine against this, which has been persistently fatal. This man knew of two cases who were, as he puts it, 'good cases for dying', and therefore good cases for trying his theory on. Both got well, began to recover within eight hours. And one of them was my re-enlisted Warwickshire man with the arm amputated, who was got out by the wounded officer and the Padre.

January 3rd.
A sergeant we took down to Havre yesterday told me of his battalion's very heavy losses. He said out of the 1400 of all ranks he came out with, there are now only 5 sergeants, 1 officer, and 72 men left. He said the young officers won't take

cover – 'they get too excited and won't listen to people who've 'ad a little experience.' One would keep putting his head out of the trench because he hadn't seen a German. 'I kept tellin' of him,' said the sergeant, 'but of course he got 'it!'

On No.— Ambulance Train (5)

WINTER ON THE TRAIN
AND IN THE TRENCHES

January 7, 1915, to February 6, 1915.

The Petit Vitesse siding—Uncomplainingness of Tommy—
Painting the train—A painful convoy—The 'Yewlan's'
watch—'Officer dressed in bandages'—Sotteville—
Versailles—The Palais Trianon—A walk at Rouen—The
German view, and the English view—'Punch'—'When you
return Conqueror'—K.'s new Army.

Thursday, January 7th.
We moved out of Boulogne about 4 a.m., and reached
Merville (with many long waits) at 2 p.m. Loaded up there,
and filled up at Hazebrouck on way back. Many cases of
influenza with high temperatures, also rheumatisms and bad
feet, very few wounded. When they got the khaki hankies
they said, 'Khaki? that's extra!'

9.30 p.m. We have 318 on board this time, including four
enterics, four diphtherias, and eighteen convalescent scarlets (who
caught it from their billet). A quiet-looking little man has a very
fine new German officer's helmet and sword. 'He gave it to me,'
he said. 'I had shot him through the lung. I did the wound up as
best I could and tried to save him, but he died. He was coming for

me with his sword.' Seems funny to first shoot a man and then try to mop it up. The Germans don't; they finish you off.

An officer on the train told me how another officer and twenty-five men were told off to go and take a new trench which had been dug in the night. Instead of the few they expected they found it packed with Germans, all asleep. 'It's not a pretty story,' he said, 'but you can't go first and tell them you're coming when you are outnumbered three to one.' They had to bayonet every one of those sleeping Germans, and killed every one without losing a man.

All my half of the train had khaki hankies and sweets; they simply loved them. They are all, except the infectious cases, just out of the trenches, and such things make them absurdly happy; you would hardly believe it. I am keeping the writing-cases and bull's-eyes for the next lot. There were just enough mufflers to muffle the chilly necks of those who hadn't already got them.

The wet has outwetted itself all day – it must be a record flood everywhere. We shall not unload to-night, so I had better think about turning in, as I have the third watch at 4 a.m.

I found some lovely eau-de-Cologne and shampoo powders from R. among the mufflers, and a pet aluminium candlestick from G. Such things give a Sister on an A.T. absurd pleasure; you'd hardly believe it.

Friday, January 8th.
Still pouring. We unloaded by 9 a.m., got our mail in. My wardmaster was so drunk to-night that the Q.M.S. had to send for the O.C. And he had just got his corporal's stripe. He was a particular ally of mine and was in South Africa.

We are in that foulest of all homes for lost trains to-day, the Petit Vitesse siding out of B. station, with the filth of all the ages around, about, and below us. You have to shut your window to keep out the smell of burning garbage and other horrors.

It is nearly three months since I sat in a chair, except at meals, and that is only a flap-down seat, or saw a fire, except the pails of coke the Tommies have on the lines.

I expect we shall be off again to-night somewhere.

Saturday, January 9th.

Did you see the H.A.C.'s story of the frozen Tommy who asked them to warm his hands, and then seeing they were on their way to his trench hastily explained that he was all right – only a bit numb. One thing one notices about them is that they have an enormous tolerance for each other and never seem to want to quarrel. They take infinite pains in the night not to wake each other in moving over the heaps of legs and arms sprawled everywhere, and will keep in cramped positions for hours rather than risk touching someone else's painful feet or hand. If you want to improve matters they say, 'I shall be all right, Sister, it might jog his foot.' They never let you miss any one out in giving things round, and always call your attention to any one they think needs it, but not to themselves. It is very funny how they won't fuss about themselves, and in consequence you often find things out too late. Last journey a man with asthma and bronchitis was, unfortunately as it turned out, given a top bunk, as he was considered too bad to be a sitting-up case. At 6 a.m. I found him looking very tired and miserable sitting on the edge; 'I can't lie down,' he said, 'with this cough.' When I put him in a sitting-up corner below, he said, 'I could a'slep' all night like this!' It had never occurred to him to ask to be changed. They get so used to discomfort that they 'stay put' and never utter. We had missed his distress (in the 318 we had on board), and they were sleeping on the floors of the corridors, so the middle bunks were very difficult to get at. Any of them would have changed with him. This happens several times on every journey, but you can't get them to fuss. The Germans and the Sikhs begin to clamour for something directly they are on the train, and keep it up till they go off.

Another typical instance (though not a pretty one) of Tommy's reluctance to complain occurred on the last journey. I came on one compartment full, busily engaged in collecting J.J.'s off one man in the middle, with a candle to see by. His blanket, I found, was swarming, and it was ours, not his, one of a lot taken on at Rouen as 'disinfected'! (For one ghastly moment I thought it might be the compartment where I'd spent a good half-hour doing up their feet, but it wasn't.) I had the blanket hurled out of the window, and they then slept. But they weren't going to complain about it.

There was one jovial old boy of 60 with rows of ribbons. He had three sons in the Army, and when they went 'he wasn't going to be left behind', so he re-enlisted.

Sunday, January 10th.
Woke up at Bailleul, sun shining for once, and everything – floods and all – looking lovely all the way down. Loaded up early and got down to B. by 4 p.m. to hear that we are to go on to Rouen – another all-night touch. We have put off the fourteen worst cases at B., and are now on our way to R. This is the first time we have shipped Canadians, P.P.C.L.I., the only regiment as yet in the fighting line. They are oldish men who have nearly all seen service before, many in South Africa.

Lots more wounded this time. Some S.L.I. got badly caught in a wood; they've just come from India.

When I took the Devonshire toffee round, a little doubtful whether the H.A.C.'s would not be too grand for it, one of them started up, 'Oh, by George, not really!'

We have a boy on board with no wound and no disease, but quite mad, poor boy; he has to have a special orderly on him.

Monday morning, January 11th, Rouen.
The approach to Rouen at six o'clock on a pitch-dark, wet, and starlight morning, with the lights twinkling on the hills and on the river, and in the old wet streets, is a beautiful sight.

My mad boy has been very quiet all night.

Tuesday, January 12th.
At S. all day. By some mistake it hasn't rained all day, so we took the opportunity to get on with painting the train. We worked all the morning and afternoon and got a lot done, and it looks very smart: huge red crosses on white squares in the middle of each coach, and the number of the ward in figures a foot long at each end: this on both sides of the coaches. We

have done not quite half the coaches, and are praying that it won't rain before it dries; if it does, the result is pitiable. The orderlies have been shining up the brass rails and paraffining the outside of the train, and have also played and won a football match against No. 1 A.T.

Wednesday, January 13th.
Woke at Abbeville; now on the way to Boulogne, where I hope we shall have time to get mails.

5 p.m. We went through Boulogne without stopping, and got no mails in consequence; nor could we pick up P., who has been on ninety-six hours' leave. We have been on the move practically without stopping since 11 p.m. last night, and are just getting to Béthune, the place we went to two days after Christmas, where we were quite near the guns, and went over the Cl. H. which had been shelled. Expect to take wounded up here. The country is wetter than ever – it looks one vast swamp. Of course the rain has spoilt our lovely paint!

Thursday, January 14th.
We picked up a load in the dark and wet, with some very badly wounded, who kept us busy from 6 p.m. to 4 a.m. without stopping. Some were caked with mud exactly to their necks! One told me he got hit trying to dig out three of his section who were half buried by an exploded coal-box. When he got hit, they were left, and eventually got finished by our own guns. Another lot of eleven were buried likewise, and are there still, but were all killed instantaneously. One man with part of his stomach blown away and his right thigh smashed was trying to get a corporal of his regiment in, but the corporal died when he got there, and he got it as well. He was smiling and thanking all night, and saying how comfortable he was. Another we had to put off at St Omer, on the off chance of saving his life. He was made happy by two tangerine oranges.

Many of the sitting-ups have no voice, and they cough all night. We unloaded this morning, got a sleep this afternoon, and are now, 5 p.m., on our way up again. The Clearing Hospitals

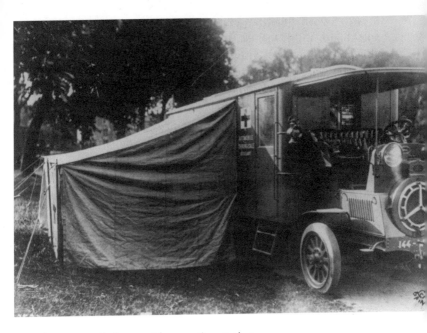

A motor ambulance with operating station.

are overflowing as of old, and like the Field Ambulances have more than they can cope with. We have to re-dress the septic things with H_2O_2, which keeps them going till they can be specially treated at the base. Some of the enterics are very bad: train journeys are not ideal treatment for enteric hæmorrhage, but it has to be done. Two of my orderlies are very good with them, and take great care of their mouths, and know how to feed them. It is a great anxiety when a great hulking G.D.O. (General Duty Orderly, not a Nursing Orderly) has to take his turn on night duty with the badly wounded.

It is time the sun shone somewhere – but it will surely, later on.

Friday, January 15th.
We got to Bailleul too late last night for loading, and went

thankfully to bed instead. Now, 3.30 p.m., nearly back at B., but expect to be sent on to Rouen: most sick this time, and bad feet, not exactly frost-bite, but swollen and discoloured from the wet. One of my enterics is a Field Ambulance boy, with a temp. of 105, and he only 'went sick' yesterday. How awful he must have felt on duty. He says his body feels 'four sizes too big for him'.

It is a mild day, sunny in parts, and not wet.

Still Friday, January 15th.

We unloaded at 6 p.m. at B., and are to start off again at 4.15 a.m.; business is brisk just now; this last lot only had mostly minor ailments, besides the enterics and the woundeds.

The French Major has had a letter from his wife at last, they are with the Germans, but quite well. We drank their health to-night in special port and champagne! and had Christmas pudding with sauce d'Enfer, as the lighted brandy was called! But we are all going to bed, not *ivrés* I'm glad to tell you. This going up by night and down by day is much the least tiring way, as we can undress and have a real night in bed.

Later. Hazebrouck. We have been out, but couldn't get as far as No.— Cl. H. (where I find T. is), as the R.T.O. said we might be going on at 11.30.

We came across an anti-aircraft gun pointing to the sky, on a little hill. The gunner officer in charge of it seemed very pleased to see us, as he is alone all day. (He walks up and down the road a certain distance, dropping stones out of his pocket at each turning, and clears out the surrounding drain-pipes to drain his bit of swamp, as his amusements.)

He showed us his two kinds of 12 lb. shells, high explosives and shrapnel. The high explosive frightens the enemy aeroplane away by its terrific bang, he says: our own airmen say they don't mind the shrapnel. He says you can't distinguish between one kind of French aeroplane and the Germans until they are close enough over you to see the colours underneath, and then it may be too late to fire. 'I'm terrified of bringing down a French aeroplane,' he said. He was a most cheerful, ruddy, fit-looking boy.

9 P.M. Another train full, and nearing Boulogne; a supply train full of minor cases came down just before us from the same place, where we've been three days running. The two Clearing Hospitals up there are working at awful high pressure – filling in from Field Ambulances, and emptying into the trains. All cases now have to go through the Clearing Hospitals for classification and diagnosis and dressings, but it is of a sketchy character, as you may imagine. They are all swarming with J.J.'s, even the officers. One of the officers is wounded in the head, shoulder, stomach, both arms, and both feet. A boy in my wards, with a baby face, showed me a beautiful silver, enamelled and engraved watch he got off a 'Yewlan'; he was treasuring it in his belt 'to take home to Mother'. I asked him if the Yewlan was dead. 'Oh yes,' he said, his face lighting up with glee; 'we shot him. He was like a pepper-pot when we got to him.' Isn't it horrible? And like the boy in *Punch*, he'd never killed anybody before he went to France. I wonder what 'Mother' will say to his cheerful little story.

I have been busy bursting a bad quinsy with inhalers and fomentations. After a few hours he could sing Tipperary and drink a bottle of stout!

There are two Volunteer shop-boys from a London Territorial Regiment, who call me 'Madam' from force of habit.

Sunday, January 17th.

We didn't unload at Boulogne last night, and are still (11 a.m.) taking them on to Étretat, a lovely place on the coast, about ten miles north of Havre. The hospital there is my old No.— General Hospital, that I mobilised with, so it will be very jolly to see them all again.

We are going through most lovely country on a clear sunny morning, and none of the patients are causing any anxiety, so it is an extremely pleasant journey, and we shall have a good rest on the way back.

3 p.m. Just as I was beginning to forget there were such things as trenches and shrapnel and snipers, they told me a horrible story of two Camerons who got stuck in the mud and sucked down to

their shoulders. They took an hour and a half getting one out, and just as they said to the other, 'All right, Jock, we'll have you out in a minute,' he threw back his head and laughed, and in doing so got sucked right under, and is there still. They said there was no sort of possibility of getting him out; it was like a quicksand.

One told me – not as such a very sensational fact – that he went for eleven weeks without taking off his clothes, *or a wash*, and then he had a hot bath and a change of everything. He remarked that he had to scrape himself with a knife.

We have been travelling all day, and shan't get to Étretat till about 7 p.m. It is a mercy we got our bad cases off at Boulogne – pneumonias, enterics, two s.f.'s, and some badly wounded, including the officer dressed in bandages all over. He was such a nice boy. When he was put into clean pyjamas, and had a clean hanky with eau-de-Cologne, he said, 'By Jove, it's worth getting hit for this, after the smells of dead horses, dead men, and dead everything.' He said no one could get into Messines, where there is only one house left standing, because of the unburied dead lying about. He couldn't move his arms, but he loved being fed with pigs of tangerine orange, and, like so many, he was chiefly concerned with 'giving so much trouble'. He looked awfully ill, but seldom stopped smiling. Of such are the Kingdom of Heaven.

Later. On way to Havre. These are all bound for home and have been in hospital some time. They are clean, shaved, clothed, fed, and convalescent. Most of the lying-downs are recovering from severe wounds of weeks back. It is quite new even to see them at that stage, instead of the condition we usually get them in. Some are the same ones we brought down from Béthune three weeks ago.

One man was in a dug-out going about twenty feet back from the trench, with sixteen others, taking cover from our howitzers and also from the enemy's. The cultivated ground is so soft with the wet that it easily gives, and the bursting of one of our shells close by drove the roof in and buried these seventeen – four were killed and eleven injured by it, but only two were got out alive, and they were abandoned as dead. However, a rescue party of six faced the enemy shells above ground and tried to get them out. In doing this two were killed and two wounded. The other two went on with it. My man and another man were pinned down by beams – the other had his face clear, but mine hadn't, though he could hear the picks above him. He gave up all hopes of getting out, but the other man when rescued said he thought this one was still alive, and then got him out unconscious. When he came to he was in hospital in a chapel, and it took him a long time to realise he was alive. 'They generally take you into chapel before they bury you,' he said, 'but I told 'em they done it the wrong way round with me. That was the worst mess ever I got into in this War,' he finished up.

Wednesday, January 20th, Sotteville.
The others have all been out, but I've been a bit lazy and stayed in, washed my hair and mended my clothes. This place is looking awfully pretty to-day, because all the fields are flooded between us and the long line of high hills about a mile away, and it looks like a huge lake with the trees reflected in it. No orders to move, as usual. Ambulance trains travel as 'specials' in a 'marche', which means a gap in the timetable. There are only about two marches in twenty-four hours, and the R.T.O.'s have to fit the A.T.'s in to one or other of these marches when orders come that No.— A.T. is wanted. We do not get final orders of where our destination is till we get to Hazebrouck or St Omer. We have been six days without a mail now, and have taken loads to Étretat and to Havre.

Thursday, January 21st.
We were not a whole day at Sotteville for once: moved out early this morning and are still travelling, 9 p.m., between Abbeville and Boulogne. It has been a specially slow journey, and, alas! we didn't go by Amiens: the only time we might have, by daylight. Beauvais has a fine Cathedral from the outside. I believe we are to go straight on from Boulogne, so we may not get our six days' mail, alas!
Friday, January 22nd.

We didn't get in to B. till midnight, too late to get mails, and left early this morning. At Calais it was discovered that the kitchen had been left behind, in shunting a store waggon, so we have been hung up all day waiting for it at St Omer. Went for a walk. It is a most interesting place to walk about in, swarming with every kind of war material, and the grey towers of the two Cathedrals looked lovely in a blue sky. Such a dazzling day: we were able to get on with painting the train, which is breaking out into the most marvellous labelling, the orderlies competing with each other. But when at 6 p.m. it seemed the day would never end, No.— A.T. steamed up with our kitchen tacked on, and in the kitchen was the mail-bag – joy of joys!

We have just got to Bailleul, 10.30 p.m.: a few guns banging. We are wondering if we shall clear the Cl. hospitals to-night or wait till morning: depends if they are expecting convoys in to-night and are full.

11 p.m. P. and I, fully rigged for night duty, have just been gloomily exploring the perfectly silent and empty station and street, wondering when the motor ambulances would begin to roll up, when B—— hailed us from the train with '8 o'clock to-morrow morning, you two sillies, and the Major's in bed!' so now we can turn in, and load up happily by daylight, and it's my turn for the lying down, thank goodness, or rather the Liers, as they are called.

Saturday, January 23rd.
Another blue, sunny, frosty morning. Loading up this morning was hard to attend to, as a thrilling Taube chase was going on overhead, the sky peppered with bursting shells, and aeroplanes buzzing around: didn't bring it down though.

The train is full of very painful feet: like a form of large burning chilblain all over the foot, and you can't do anything for them, poor lambs.

Still Saturday, January 23rd.
This is our first journey to Versailles. My only acquaintance with it was on the way up from Le Mans to Villeneuve to join this train.

Two kind sisters, living in a sort of little ticket office in the middle of the line, washed and fed me at 6 a.m. in between two trains, but I saw nothing of the glories of Versailles – hope to to-morrow.

I don't think the men will get much sleep, their feet are too bad, but we are going to give them a good chance with drugs, the last thing. We shall do the night in three watches.

Sunday, January 24th, 5 a.m., *Versailles.*
They've had a pretty good night most of them. If you see any compartment, say six sitters and two top-liers showing signs of being near the end of their tether, with bad feet and long hours of the train, you have only to say cheerfully, 'How are you getting on in this dug-out?' for every man to brighten visibly, and there is a chorus of 'If our dug-outs was like this I reckon we shouldn't want no relievin'!' and a burst of wit and merriment follows. You can try it all down the train; it never fails.

They are all in 1st class coaches, not 3rds or 2nds.

9.30 a.m. They have only four M.A.'s, and the hospital is 1-1/2 miles off, so all our 366 limping, muddy scarecrows are not off yet. There is a mist and a piercing north wind, and lots of mud. The A.T.'s do so much bringing the British Army from the field that I hope some other trains are busy bringing the British Army to the field, or there can't be many left in the field.

They told me another story of a man in the Royal Scots who was sunk in mud up to his shoulders, and the officer offered a canteen of rum and a sovereign to the first man who could get him out. For five hours thirteen men were digging for him, but it filled up always as they dug, and when they got him out he died.

6 p.m. Just getting to Rouen, probably to load for Havre. They do keep us moving. We just had time to go and see the Palais Trianon with the French Sergeant (who is nearly a gentleman, and an artist). Is there anything else quite like it anywhere else? It was *défense d'entrer*, so we only wandered round the grounds and looked in at the windows, down the avenues and round the ponds and hundreds of statues, and went up the great *escalier*. Louis Quatorze certainly did himself proud.

It was a long way to go, and we were walking for hours till we got dog-tired after the long load from Bailleul, and after lunch retired firmly on to our beds. I don't think we shall take patients on to-night.

Monday, January 25th.
We have been at Sotteville all day; had time to read last week's *Times* – an exceptionally interesting lot.

Have just had orders to load up at Rouen for Havre to-morrow; then I hope we shall go back to Boulogne. We have not stayed more than an hour or two in Boulogne since January 9th – that is, for seventeen days; but we've managed to just pick up our mails every few days while unloading the bad cases. We ought to get back there for a mail on Thursday.

We have taken down a good many Northamptons lately. They seem an exceptionally seasoned and intelligent lot, and have been through the thick of everything since Mons.

Did I tell you that in one place (I don't suppose it is the same all along the line) they are doing forty-eight hours in the trenches, followed by forty-eight hours back in the billets (barns, &c.) for six times, and then twelve days' rest, when they get themselves and their rifles cleaned; they have armourers' shops for this.

They nearly all say that only the men who are quite certain they never will get back, say they want to. If any others say it, 'Well, they're liars.' But for all that, you do find one here and there who means it. One Canadian asked how long he'd be sick with his feet. 'I want to get back to the regiment,' he said. They seem rather out of it with the Tommies, some of them.

Just had a grand hot bath from a passing engine in exchange for chocolate.

We shall have a quiet night to-night. Sotteville is the quietest place we ever sleep in; there is no squealing of whistles and shouting of French railwaymen as in all the big stations. Last night they were shunting and jigging us about all night between Rouen and Sotteville. Slow bumping over hundreds of points is much worse to sleep in than fast travelling. In either case you wake whenever you pull up or start off. But we shall miss the train when we get into a dull hotel bedroom or a billet, or perhaps a tent. My month at Le Mans in Madame's beautiful French bed was the one luxury I've struck so far.

Tuesday, 26th January.
A dazzling blue spring day. As we were not going in to load at Rouen till 3 p.m., we went for the most glorious walk in this country. We crossed the ferry over the Seine to the foot of the steep high line of hills which eventually overlooks Rouen, and climbed up to the top by a lovely winding woody path in the sun. (The boatman congratulated us on the sinking of the *Blücher*, as a naval man, I suppose.) 'Who said War?' said P. while we were waiting on the shingle for the boat; it did seem very remote. At the top we got to the Church of Le Bon Secours, which is in a very fine position with a marvellous view. We had some lovely cider in a very clean pub with a garden, and then took the tram down a very steep track into Rouen. I was standing in the front of the tram for the view over Rouen, which was dazzling, with the spires and the river and the bridges, when we turned a sharp corner and smashed bang into a market-cart coming up our track. For the moment one thought the man and woman and the horse must be done for; the horse disappeared under the tram, and there arose such a screaming that the three Tommies and I fell over each other trying to get out to the rescue. When we did we found the man and woman had been luckily shot out clear of the tram, except that the man's hand was torn, and the old woman was frantically screaming, 'Mon cheval, mon cheval, mon cheval,' at least a hundred times without stopping. The others were out by this time and the two tram people, and the French clack went on at its top speed, while P. and the Tommies and a very clever old woman out of the tram tried to cut the horse clear of the broken cart, and I did up the man's hand with our hankies; the only one concerned least was the horse, who kept quiet with its legs mixed up in the tram. At last the tram succeeded in moving clear of the horse without hurting it, and it was got up smiling after all. The outside old woman went on

picking up the fish and the harness, &c., the man was taken off to have his hand bathed, and the poor old woman of the cart stopped screaming 'Mon cheval, mon cheval,' and went off to have a drink, and we walked on and found a train at Rouen. That sort of thing is always happening in France.

I hope the overworked people at the heads of the various departments of the British Army realise how the men appreciate what they try and do for them in the trenches. If you ask what the billets are like, they say, 'Barns and suchlike; they do the best they can for us.' If you ask if the trench conditions are as bad for the Germans, they say, 'They're worse off; they ain't looked after like what we are.'

9.30 p.m. On way to Havre. I was just going to say that from the Seine to Le Havre there is nothing to report, when I came across a young educated German in my wards with his left leg off from the hip, and his right from below the knee, and a bad shell wound in his arm, all healed now, done at Ypres on 24th October. And I had an hour's most thrilling and heated conversation with him in German. He was very down on the English Sisters in hospital, because he says they hated him and didn't treat him like the rest. I said that was because they couldn't forget what his regiment (Bavarians) had done to the Belgian women and children and old men, and the French. And he said *he* couldn't forget how the Belgian women had put out the eyes of the German wounded at Liège and thrown boiling water on them. I said they were driven to it. I asked him a lot of straight questions about Germany and the War, and he answered equally straight. He said they had food in Germany for ten years, and that they had ten million men, and that all the present students would be in the Army later on, and that practically the supply could never stop. And I said that however long they could go on, in the end there would be no more Germany because she was up against five nations. He said no man has any fear of a Russian soldier, and that though they were slow over it they would get Paris, but not London except by Zeppelins; he admitted that it would be *sehr schwer* to land troops in England, and that our Navy was the best, but we had so few soldiers, they hardly counted! He got very excited over the Zeppelins. I asked why the Germans hated the English, and he said, 'In Berlin we do not speak of the English at all(!!!); it is the French and the Russians we hate.' He said the Turks were no good *zu helfen*, and Austria not much better. He was very down on Belgium for resisting in the first place! and said the *Schuld* was with France and Russia. They were very much astonished when England didn't remain neutral! He had the cheek to say that three German soldiers were as good as twenty English, so I assured him that five English could do for fifty Germans, and went on explaining carefully to him how there could be no more Germany in the end because the right must win! and he said, 'So you say in England, but we know otherwise in Deutschland, and I am a German.' So as I am an English we had to agree to differ. His faith in his *Vaterland* nearly made him cry and must have given him a temperature. I felt quite used up afterwards. He is fast asleep now. There is also an old soldier of sixty-three who says General French and General Smith-Dorrien photographed him as the oldest soldier in the British Army. He has four sons in it, one killed, two wounded. He was with General Low in the Chitral Expedition, and is called Donald Macdonald, of the K.O.S.B.'s. 'Unfortunately I was reduced to the ranks for being drunk the other day,' he said gaily. 'But the Captain he said, "Don't lose 'eart, Macdonald, you'll get it all back."'

Wednesday, January 27th.
They have found a way of warming our quarters when we have not an engine on. I don't know what we should have done without it to-day; it is icy cold. Mails to-morrow, hurrah! Going to turn in early.

Thursday, January 28th.
Got to Boulogne this morning. Have been getting stores in and repairs done; expect to be sent up any time. Sharp frost and cold wind.

Friday, January 29th.
One of those difficult-to-bear days; hung up all day at a place

beyond St Omer, listening to guns, and doing nothing when there's so much to be done. The line is probably too busy to let us up. It happens to be a dazzling blue day, which must be wiping off 50 per cent of the horrors of the Front. The other 50 per cent is what they are out for, and see the meaning of.

We are to go on in an hour's time, 'destination unknown'.

Saturday, January 30th.
We got up to Merville at one o'clock last night, and loaded up only forty-five, and are now just going to load up again at a place on the way back. We have been completely done out of the La Bassée business; haven't been near it. No.— Cl. H. that we saw on December 27th, where S.C. and two more of my No.— G.H. friends were, had to be evacuated in a hurry, as several orderlies were killed in the shelling.

One of my badly woundeds says 'the Major' (whose servant he has been for four years) asked him to make up the fire in his dug-out, while he went to the other end of the trench. While he was doing the fire a shell burst over the dug-out and a bit went through his left leg and touched his right. If the Major had been sitting in his chair where he was a minute before, his head would have been blown off. He said, 'When the Major came back and found me, he drove everybody else away and stayed with me all day, and made me cocoa, and at night carried my stretcher himself and took me right to Headquarters.' His eyes shine when he talks of 'the Major', and he seems so proud he got it instead.

I asked a boy in the sitting-ups what was the matter with him. 'Too small,' he said. Another said, 'Too young'; he was aged fifteen, in the Black Watch.

A young monkey, badly wounded in hand and throat (lighting a cigarette – the shatter to his hand saved worse destruction to his throat, though bad enough as it is), after we'd settled him in, fixed his eye on me and said, 'Are you going to be in here along of us all the way?' 'Yes,' I said. 'That's a good job,' and he is taking good care to get his money's worth, I can tell you.

Some of them are roaring at the man in *Punch* who made a

gallant attempt to do justice to all his Xmas presents at once. There is a sergeant-major of the Royal Scots very indignant at having been made to go sick with bad feet. Any attempt to fuss over him is met with 'I need no attention whatever, thank you, Sister. I feel more like apologising for being in here. Only five weeks of active service,' he growled.

The latest Franco-British idea is to Arras the Boches till they Argonne!

Sunday, January 31st.
We did go on to Rouen. B. is full to the brim. We have only unloaded at B. three times since Christmas.

I'm beginning to think we waste a lot of sympathy on the poor wounded rocking in a train all night after being on it all day. One of mine with a bullet still in his chest, and some pneumonia, who seemed very ill when he was put on at Merville, said this morning he felt a lot better and had had the best night for five days! And my fidgety boy with the wound in his throat made a terrible fuss at being put off at Boulogne when he found he was the only one in his compartment to go and that I wasn't going with him.

I had the easy watch last night because of my cold, and went to bed at 1 A.M.; got a hot bath this morning, and lay low all day till a stroll between the Seine and the floods after tea (Sotteville). There are four trains waiting here, and the C.S.'s have been skating on the floods. We move on at 1 o'clock to-night. No.— A.T. had a bomb dropped each side of their train at Bailleul, but they didn't explode.

The French instruction books have come, and I am going to start the French class for the men on the train; they are very keen to learn, chiefly, I think, to make a little more running with the French girls at the various stopping places.

Two officers last night were awfully sick at not being taken off at B., but I think they'll get home from Rouen. One said he must get home, if only for ten minutes, to feel he was out of France.

Wednesday, February 3rd.
Moved on last night, and woke up at Bailleul. Some badly

wounded on the train, but not on my half.

On the other beat, beyond Rouen, the honeysuckle is in leaf, the catkins are out, and the woods are full of buds. What a difference it will make when spring comes. On this side it is all canals, bogs, and pollards, and the eternal mud.

We found pinned on a sock from a London school child, 'Whosoever receives this, when you return conqueror, drop me a line,' and then her name and address!

Thursday, February 4th.
For once we unloaded at B. and went to bed instead of taking them on all night to Rouen.

Moved out of B. at 5 a.m., breakfast at St O., where we nearly got left behind strolling on the line during a wait. We are going to Merville in the mining district where L. is.

3 p.m. We have just taken on about seventy Indians, mostly sick, some badly wounded. They are much cleaner than they used to be, in clothes, but not, alas! in habits. Aeroplanes are chasing a Taube overhead, but it is not being shelled. Guns are making a good noise all round. We are waiting for a convoy of British now.

It is a lovely afternoon.

The guns were shaking the train just now; one big bang made us all pop our heads out of the window to look for the bomb, but it wasn't a bomb. A rosy-faced white-haired Colonel here just came up to me and said, 'You've brought us more firing this afternoon than we've heard for a long time.'

We are filling up with British wounded now on the other half of the train. It is getting late, and we shan't unload to-night.

Later. We were hours loading up because all the motor drivers are down with flu, and there were only two available. The rest are all busy bringing wounded in to the Clearing Hospital.

The spell of having the train full of slight medical cases and bad feet seems to be over, and wounded are coming on again.

Three of my sitting-up Indians have temperatures of 104, so you can imagine what the lying-downs are like. They are very

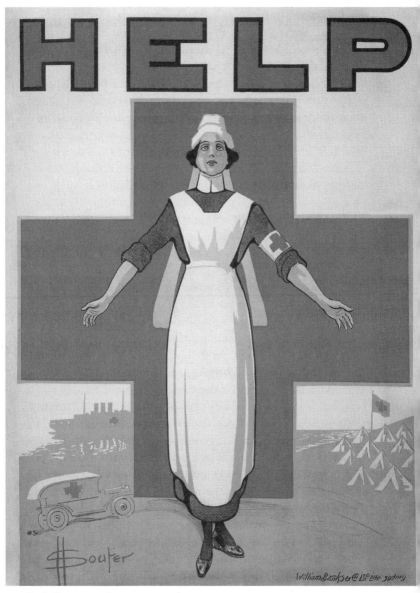

Red Cross recruitment poster for nurses.

anxious cases to look after, partly because they are another race and partly because they can't explain their wants, and they seem to want to be let die quietly in a corner rather than fall in with your notions of their comfort.

At Bailleul on our last journey we took on a heavenly white puppy just old enough to lap, quite wee and white and fat. He cries when he wants to be nursed, and barks in a lovely falsetto when he wants to play, and waddles after our feet when we take him for a walk, but he likes being carried best.

Some Tommies on a truck at Railhead brought him up for us; they adore his little mother and two brothers.

Friday, February 5th, Boulogne.
We did get in late last night, and got to bed at 1 a.m. They are unloading during the night again now, and also loading up at night.

One boy last night had lost his right hand; his left arm and leg were wounded, and both his eyes. 'Yes, I've got more than my share,' he said, 'but I'll get over it all right.' I didn't happen to answer for a minute, and in a changed voice he said, 'Shan't I? shan't I?' Of course I assured him he'd get quite well, and that he was ticketed to go straight to an eye specialist. 'Thank God for that,' he said, as if the eye specialist had already cured him, but it is doubtful if any eye specialist will save his eyes.

To-day has been a record day of brilliant sun, blue sky and warm air, and it has transformed the muddy, sloppy, dingy Boulogne of the last two months into something more like Cornwall. We couldn't stop on the train (there were no orders likely), in spite of being tired, but went in the town in the morning, and on the long stone pier in the afternoon, and then to tea at the buffet at the Maritime (where you have tea with real milk and fresh butter, and jam not out of a tin, and a tablecloth, and a china cup—luxuries beyond description). On the pier there were gulls, and a sunny sort of salt wind and big waves breaking, and a glorious view of the steep little town piled up in layers above the harbour, which is packed with shipping.

Rouen – Neuve Chapelle – St Eloi

February 7, 1915, to March 31, 1915

The Indians—St Omer—The Victoria League—Poperinghe—
A bad load—Left behind—Rouen again—An 'off' spell—*En
route* to Étretat—Sotteville—Neuve Chapelle—St Eloi—The
Indians—Spring in N.W. France—The Convalescent Home—
Kitchener's boys.

Sunday, February 7th.
This is a little out-of-the-way town called Blendecque, rather in
a hollow. No.— A.T. has been here before, and the natives look
at us as if we were Boches. There are 250 R.E. inhabiting a long
truck-train here. We have given them all our mufflers and mittens;
they had none, and the officer has had our officers to tea with him.
Our men have played a football match with them – drawn.

We went for a splendid walk this morning up hill to a pine
wood bordered by a moor with whins. I've now got in my
bunky-hole (it is not quite six feet square) a polypod fern,
a plate of moss, a pot of white hyacinths, and also catkins,
violets, and mimosa!

I suppose we shall move on to-night if there is a marche.

Many hundreds of French cavalry passed across the bridge

over this cutting this morning: they looked so jolly.

One of the staff who has been to Woolwich on leave says that K.'s new army there is extraordinarily promising and keen. So far we have only heard good of those out here, from the old hands who've come across them.

9.45 p.m. We are just getting to the place where all the fighting is – La Bassée way. Probably we shall load up with wounded to-night. There's a great flare some way off that looks like the burning villages we used to see round Ypres. It is a very dark night.

Monday morning, February 8th.
We stood by last night, and are just going to load now. All is quiet here. Said to have been nothing happening the last few days.

7 p.m. Nearing B. We've had a very muddly day, taking on at four different places. I have a coach full of Indians. They have been teaching me some more Hindustani. Some of them suddenly began to say their prayers at sunset. They spread a small mat in front of them, knelt down, and became very busy 'knockin' 'oles in the floor with their 'eads', as the orderly describes it.

We have a lot of woundeds from Saturday's fighting. They took three German trenches, and got in with the bayonet until they were 'treading' on dead Germans! The wounded sitting-ups are frightfully proud of it. After their personal reminiscences you feel as if you'd been jabbing Germans yourself. They say they 'lose their minds' in the charge, and couldn't do it if they stopped to think, 'because they're feelin' men, same as us,' one said.

A corporal on his way back to the Front from taking some people down to St O. under a guard saw one of his pals at the window in our train. He leaped up and said, 'I wish to God I could get chilblains and come down with you.' This to an indignant man with a shrapnel wound!

I've got five bad cases of measles, with high temperatures and throats.

Tuesday, February 9th.
Again they unloaded us at B. last night, and we are now, 11 a.m., on our way up again. The Indians I had were a very interesting

lot. The race differences seem more striking the better you get to know them. The Gurkhas seem to be more like Tommies in temperament and expression, and all the Mussulmans and the best of the Sikhs and Jats might be Princes and Prime Ministers in dignity, feature, and manners. When a Sikh refuses a cigarette (if you are silly enough to offer him one) he does it with a gesture that makes you feel like a housemaid who ought to have known better. The beautiful Mussulmans smile and salaam and say Merbani, however ill they are, if you happen to hit upon something they like. They all make a terrible fuss over their kit and their puggarees and their belongings, and refuse to budge without them.

Sister M. found her orders to leave when we got in, but she doesn't know where she is going. So after this trip we shall be three again, which is a blessing, as there are not enough wards for four, and no one likes giving any up. It also gives us a spare bunk to store our warehouses of parcels for men, which entirely overflow our own dug-outs. As soon as you've given out one lot, another bale arrives.

We have had every kind of infectious disease to nurse in this war, except smallpox. The Infectious Ward is one of mine, and we've had enteric, scarlet fever, measles, mumps, and diphtheria.

7 p.m. We got to the new place where we wait for a marche, just at tea-time, and we had a grand walk up to the moor, where you can see half over France each way. There is a travelling wireless station up there. Each pole has its receiver in a big grey motor-lorry by the roadside, where they live and sleep. The road wound down to a little curly village with a beautiful old grey church. On the top of the moor on the way back it was dark, and the flash signals were morsing away to each other from the different hills. It reminded me of the big forts on the kopjes round Pretoria.

I had my first French class this afternoon at St Omer, in the men's mess truck. There were seventeen, including the Quartermaster-Sergeant and the cook's boy. I'd got a small blackboard in Boulogne, and they all had notebooks, and the Q.M.S. had arranged it very nicely. They were very keen, and got on at a great pace. They weren't a bit shy over trying to pronounce, and will I think make good progress. They have a great pull over men of their class in England, by their opportunities of listening to French spoken by the French, such a totally different language to French spoken by most English people. My instruction book is Hugo's, which is a lightning method compared to the usual school-books. They are doing exercises for me for next time.

Wednesday, February 10th, 9 p.m.
We woke at Merville after a particularly rocky, noisy night journey, and loaded up there with woundeds and sick, also Indians (but not in my wards for once). My *blessés* kept me busy till the moment we unloaded this evening at B., and I had not time to hear much about their doings. One extraordinarily sporting boy had a wound right through his neck, involving his swallowing. It took about half an hour to give him a feed, through a tube, but he stuck it, smiling all the time.

Another older man was shot in the stomach, and looked as if he wouldn't get over it. He told me he'd already been in hospital eight weeks, shot in the head at the Aisne. I said what hard luck to have to go through it again. 'It's got to be done,' he said. 'I didn't give it a thought. I think I shall get over this,' he said, 'but I don't want to go back a third time.' He has a wife and three children in Ireland.

We are to move up again at 4 a.m. Just had dinner (soup, boiled beef as tough as a cable, and ration cheese and coffee), and the 'Daily Mail.'

Thursday, February 11th.
We have spent most of the day at St Omer, and got a lovely walk in this morning, along the canal, watching the big barges which take 2000 tons of beetroots for sugar.

There is a scheme on foot for fitting up these big barges as transport for the sick (this one came from Furnes) as moving Clearing Hospitals. I've been over one, in Rouen. They are not yet in use, but might be rather jolly in the summer.

It is the warmest spring day we've had. I had my second French class this afternoon again at St Omer. We are now moving on, up to Bailleul. I expect we shall take patients on this evening, and have them all night.

Friday, February 12th, 6 a.m.
We did a record loading up in fifty minutes last night, chiefly medical cases, and took eight hours to crawl to Boulogne. Now we are on the way for Havre, but shall not get there till about 10 p.m. to-night, so they will have a long day in the train.

A good many of the lying-downs are influenza, with high temperatures and no voice. It is a bore getting to B. in the night, as we miss our mails and the *Daily Mail*.

7 p.m. This is an interminable journey. Have not yet reached Rouen, and shan't get to Havre till perhaps 2 a.m. The patients are getting very weary, especially the sitting-ups. The wards of acute liers you can run like a hospital. Some of the orderlies are now getting quite keen on having their wards clean and swept, and the meals and feeds up to time, and the washings done, but it has taken weeks to bring them up to it. When they do all that well I can get on with the diets, temperatures, treatments, and dressings, &c. On the long journeys we take round at intervals smokes, chocolate, papers, hankies, &c., when we have them. The Victoria League has done me well in bales of hankies. They simply love the affectionate and admiring messages pinned on from New Zealand, and one of them always volunteers to answer them.

We shall be up in shifts again to-night.

We are all hoping to have a day in Rouen on the way back, for baths, hair-washing, shopping, seeing the Paymaster, and showing the new Sister the sights. For sheer beauty and interestingness it is the most endearing town; you don't know which you love best – its setting with the hills, river, and bridge, or its beautiful spires and towers and marvellous old streets and houses.

Saturday, February 13th, 2 a.m.
Still on the way to Havre! And we loaded up on Thursday. This journey is another revelation of what the British soldier

will stick without grumbling. The sitting-ups are eight in a carriage, some with painful feet, some with wounded arms, and some with coughs, rheumatism, &c., but you don't hear a word of grousing. It is only when things are prosperous and comfortable that Tommy grumbles and has grievances. Some of the liers are too ill to know how long they've been on the train. One charming Scotchman, who enlisted for K.'s Army, but was put into the Regulars because he could shoot, has just asked me to write my name and address in his little book so that he can write from England. He also says we must 'look after ourselves' and 'study our health', because there's a bad time coming, and our Country will need us! He's done his share, after an operation, and will never be able to do any more. Everything points to this Service having to put out all it can, both here and at home. Many new hospitals are being organised, and there are already hundreds.

We have a poor lunatic on board who keeps asking us to let his wife come in. The train is crawling with J.J.'s.

Saturday, 4.30 a.m.
Just seen the last stretcher off; now going to undress (first time since Wednesday night) and turn in.

Saturday, 13th February, Havre.
It is four months to-day since I joined the train. It seems much longer in some ways, and yet the days go by very quickly – even the off-days; and when the train is full the hours fly.

We went into the familiar streets this morning that we saw so much of in August, 'waiting for orders', and had a look at the sea. The train moved off at tea-time, so we had the prettiest part of the journey in a beautiful evening sunlight, lighting up the woods and hills. The palm is out, and the others saw primroses. We have also seen some snowdrops.

After a heavy journey, with two nights out of bed, you don't intend to do any letter-writing or mending or French classes, but look out of the window or sleep or read Dolly Dialogues. You always get compensation for these journeys in the longer journey back, with probably a wait at Rouen or Sotteville, and possibly another at Boulogne. We have been going up and down again very briskly this last fortnight between B. and the Back of the Front.

Sunday, 14th.
A dismal day at Sotteville; pouring cats and dogs all day, and the train cold.

Shrove Tuesday.
We were all day coming up yesterday. Got to B. in the middle of the night, and went on again to St Omer, where we woke this morning, so we missed our mails again; it will be a full week's mails when we do get them. Lovely blue sky to-day. Had a walk with Sister B. round the town, and now this afternoon we are on the way to Poperinghe, in a beaten country, where we haven't been for three months. French class due at 3 p.m. if we haven't got there by then.

We have just passed a graveyard absolutely packed with little wooden crosses.

Ash Wednesday, February 17th, 6 a.m.
We took on a very bad load of wounded at Poperinghe, more like what used to happen three months ago in the same place; they were only wounded the night before, and some the same day. The Clearing Hospital had to be cleared immediately.

We have just got to B., and are going to unload here at 8.30 a.m.

Must stop. Hope to get a week's mails to-day.

A brisk air battle between one British and one French and two Taubes was going on when we got there, and a perfect sky for it. Very high up.

A wounded major on the train was talking about the men. 'It's not a case of our leading the men; we have a job to keep up with them.'

It was a pretty sad business getting them off the train this morning; there were so many compound fractures, and no amount of contriving seemed to come between them and the jolting of the train all night. And, to add to the difficulties, it was pouring in torrents and icy cold, and the railway people refused to move the train under cover, so they went out of a warm train on to damp stretchers in an icy rain. They were nearly all in thin pyjamas, as we'd had to cut off their soaking khaki: they were practically straight from the trenches. But once clear of trains, stretchers, and motor ambulances they will be warmed, washed, fed, bedded, and their fractures set under an anæsthetic. One man had his arm blown to pieces on Monday afternoon, had it amputated on Monday night, and was put into one of our wards on Tuesday, and admitted to Base Hospital on Wednesday. But that is ticklish work.

One boy, a stretcher-bearer, with both legs severely wounded, very nearly bled to death. He was pulled round somehow. About midnight, when he was packed up in wool and hot-water bottles, &c., when I asked him how he was feeling, he said gaily, 'Quite well, delightfully warm, thank you!' We got him taken to hospital directly the train got in at 4 a.m. The others were unloaded at 9 a.m.

We are now – 5 p.m. – on our way to Étaples, probably to clear the G.H. there, either to-night or to-morrow morning. It hasn't stopped pouring all day. It took me till lunch to read my enormous mail.

Major T. has heard to-day that the French railway people want his train back again for passenger traffic, so the possibility of our all being suddenly disbanded and dispersed is hanging over us; but I believe it has been threatened before.

Thursday, February 18th.
In bed, 10 p.m. We have had a very heavy day with the woundeds again from Bailleul. We unloaded again at B. this evening, and are to go up again sometime to-night.

There is a great deal going on in our front.

There was a boy from Suffolk, of K.'s Army, in my ward who has only been out three weeks. He talked the most heavenly East Anglian – 'I was agin the barn, and that fared to hit me' – all in the right sing-song.

A sergeant of the D.C.L.I. had a fearful shell wound in his thigh, which has gone wrong, and as the trouble is too high for amputation they will have their work cut out to save his life. They were getting out of the trench for a bayonet charge, and he had just collected his men when he was hit; so the officer 'shook hands with him' and went on with the charge, leaving him and another man, wounded in the leg, in the trench. They stayed there several hours with no dressings on, sinking into the mud (can you wonder it has gone wrong?), until another man turned up and helped them out; then they *walked* to the Regimental Aid Post, 200 yards away, helped by the sound man. There they were dressed and had the anti-tetanus serum injection, and were taken by stretcher-bearers to the next Dressing Station, and thence by horse ambulance to the Field Ambulance, and then by motor ambulance to where we picked them up. There are lots of F.'s regiment wounded.

Friday, February 19th.
We left B. at 5 a.m.to-day, and were delayed all the morning farther up by one of the usual French collisions. A guard had left his end of a train and was on the engine; so he never noticed that twelve empty trucks had come uncoupled and careered down a hill, where they were run into and crumpled up by a passenger train. The guard of that one was badly injured (fractured spine), but the passengers only shaken.

At St Omer Miss M. and Major T. and I were being shown over the Khaki Train when ours moved off. There was a wild stampede; the Khaki Train had all its doors locked, and we had miles to go inside to get out. Their orderlies shouted to ours to pull the communication cord – the only way of appealing to the distant engine; so it slowed down, and we clambered breathlessly on. We are side-tracked now at the jolly place of the Moor and the Wireless Lorries; probably move on in the night.

Saturday, February 20th, 9 p.m.
We've had a very unsatisfactory day, loading up at four different places, and still on our way down. I'm just going to lie down,

to be called at 2 a.m. Now we're four: two go to bed for the whole night and the other two take the train for half the night when we have a light load, as to-day. If they are all bad cases, we have two on and two off for the two watches. We have some Indians on to-day, but most British, and not many *blessés*.

The other day a huge train of reinforcements got divided by mistake: the engine went off with all the officers, and the men had a joy-ride to themselves, invaded the cafés, where they sometimes get half poisoned, and in half an hour's time there was a big scrap among themselves, with fifty casualties. So the story runs.

A humane and fatherly orderly has just brought me a stone hot-water bottle for my feet as I write this in the rather freezing dispensary coach in the middle of the train, in between my rounds. All the worst cases and the Indians were put off at B., and the measles, mumps, and diphtherias, so there isn't much to do; some are snoring like an aeroplane.

Monday, February 22nd.
We got a short walk yesterday evening after unloading at Rouen. There was a glorious sunset over the bridge, and the lights just lighting up, and Rouen looked its beautifulest. We slept at Sotteville, and this morning Sister and I walked down the line into Rouen and saw the Paymaster and the Cathedral, and did some shopping, and had a boiled egg and real butter and tea for lunch, and came back in the tram. Sister S. is in bed with influenza.

The lengthening days and better weather are making a real difference to the gloom of things, and though there is a universal undercurrent of feeling that enormous sacrifices will have to be made, it seems to be shaping for a step farther on, and an ultimate return to sanity and peace. It is such a vast upheaval when you are in the middle of it, that you sometimes actually wonder if everyone has gone mad, or who has gone mad, that all should be grimly working, toiling, slaving, from the firing line to the base, for more Destruction, and for more highly-finished and uninterrupted Destruction, in order to get Peace. And the men who pay the cost in intimate personal and individual suffering and in death are not the men who made the war.

Wednesday, February 24th.

We have been all day in Boulogne, and move up at 8.15 this evening, which means loading up after breakfast and perhaps unloading to-morrow evening. It has given Sister S. another day to recover from her attack of influenza.

Have been busy one way and another all day, but went for a walk after tea and saw over the No.— G.H. at the Casino – a splendid place, working like clockwork. Lots of bad cases, but they all look clean and beautifully cared for and rigged up.

Thursday, February 25th.

Moved up to the place with the moor during the night. Glorious, clear, sunny morning. Couldn't leave the train for a real walk, as there were no orders.

This time last year the last thing one intended to do was to go and travel about France for six months, with occasional excursions into Belgium!

The Times sometimes comes the next day now.

9 p.m. The ways of French railways are impenetrable: in spite of orders for Bailleul before lunch, we are still here, and less than ever able to leave the train for a walk.

This is the fourth day with no patients on – the longest 'off' spell since before Christmas. It shows there's not much doing or much medical leakage.

Friday, February 26th. We loaded up this morning with a not very bad lot (mine all sitters except some enterics, a measles, and a diphtheria), and are on our way down again.

I am all ready packed to get off at B. if my leave is in Major M.'s office.

Saturday, February 27th, 9 p.m., *Hotel at Boulogne.*

All the efforts to get my seven days' leave have failed, as I thought they would.

Wednesday, March 3rd, Boulogne.

There is not a great deal to do or see here, especially on a wet day.

Friday, March 5th, 5 p.m.
On way down from Chocques – mixed lot of woundeds, medicals, Indians, and Canadians.

I have a lad of 24 with both eyes destroyed by a bullet, and there is a bad 'trachy'.
Nothing very much has been going on, but the German shells sometimes plop into the middle of a trench, and each one means a good many casualties.

10 p.m. We've had a busy day, and are not home yet.

My boy with the dressings on his head has not the slightest idea that he's got no eyes, and who is going to tell him? The pain is bad, and he has to have a lot of morphia, with a cigarette in between.

We shall probably not unload to-night, and I am to be called at 2 a.m.

The infectious ward is full with British enterics, dips., and measles, and Indian mumpies.

Saturday, March 6th, Boulogne.
Instead of being called at 2 for duty, was called at 1 to go to bed, as they unloaded us at that hour.

Last night we pulled up at Hazebrouck alongside a troop train with men, guns, and horses just out from the Midlands.

Two lads in a truck with their horses asked me for cigarettes. Luckily, thanks to the Train Comforts Fund's last whack, I had some. One said solemnly that he had a 'coosin' to avenge, and now his chance had come. They both had shining eyes, and not a rollicking but an eager excitement as they asked when the train would get 'there', and looked as if they could already see the shells and weren't afraid.

Sunday, March 7th.
We are stuck in the jolly place close to G.H.Q., but can't leave the train as there are no orders. I've been having a French class, with the wall of the truck for a blackboard, and occasional bangs from a big gun somewhere.

Tail-end of Monday, March 8th.

On way down to Étretat, where No.— G.H. is, which we shall reach to-morrow about tea-time. A load of woundeds this time; very busy all day till now (midnight), and haven't had time to hear many of their adventures. They seem to all come from a line of front where the Boches are persistently hammering to break through, and though they don't get any forrarder they cause a steady leakage. We heard guns all the while we were loading. A dressing-station five miles away had just been shelled, and a major, R.A.M.C., killed and two other R.A.M.C. officers wounded.

I have a man wounded in eight places, including a fractured elbow and a fractured skull, which has been trephined. What is left of him that hasn't stopped bullets is immensely proud of his bandages! He was one of nineteen who were in a barn when a shell came through the roof and burst inside, spitting shrapnel bullets all over them; all wounded and one killed. We have just put off an emergency case of gas gangrene, temp. 105, who came on as a sitter! They so often say after a bad dressing, 'I'm a lot of trouble to ye, Sister.'

Later. Just time for a line before I do another round and then call my relief. It is an awfully cold night.

Tuesday, March 9th, 12 noon.

We are passing through glorious country of wooded hills and valleys, with a blue sky and shining sun, and all the patients are enjoying it. It is still very cold, and there is a little snow about. They call their goatskin coats 'Teddy Bears'. One very ill boy, wounded in the lungs, who was put off at Abbeville, was wailing, 'Where's my Mary Box?' as his stretcher went out of the window. We found it, and he was happy.

Wednesday, March 10th.

We got to Étretat at about 3 p.m. yesterday after a two days' and one night load, and had time to go up to the hospital, where I saw S. The Matron was away. We only saw it at night last time, so it was jolly getting the afternoon there. The sea was a thundery blue, and the cliffs lit up yellow by the sun, and with the grey shingle it made a glorious picture to take back to the train. It had been a heavy journey with bad patients, and we were rather tired, so we didn't explore much.

We woke at Sotteville near Rouen this morning, and later in the day had a most fatiguing and much too exciting adventure over catching the train. Two of the Sisters and I walked into Rouen about 10.30, and found No.— A.T. marked up as still at Sotteville (in the R.T.O.'s office), and so concluded it would be there all day. So we did our businesses of hair-washing, Cathedral, lunch, &c., and then took the tram back to Sotteville. The train had gone! The Sotteville R.T.O. (about a mile off) told us it was due to leave Rouen loaded up for Havre at 2.36; it was then 2.15, and it was usually about three-quarters of an hour's walk up the line (we'd done it once this morning), so we made a desperate dash for it. Sister M. walks very slowly at her best, so we decided that I should sprint on and stop the train, and she and the other follow up. The Major met me near our engine, and was very kind and concerned, and went on to meet the other two. The train moved out three minutes after they got on. Never again! – we'll stick on it all day rather than have such a narrow shave.

We are full of convalescents for Havre to go straight on to the boat. They are frightfully enthusiastic about the way the British Army is looked after in this war. 'There's not much they don't get for us,' they said.

There are crowds of primroses out on the banks. Our infant R.A.M.C. (Officer's Mess) cook (a boy of about twenty, who looks sixteen and cooks beautifully) has just jumped off the train while it was going, grabbed a handful of primroses, and leapt on to the train again some coaches back. He came back panting and rosy, and said, 'I've got some for you, Sister!' We happened not to be going fast, but there was no question of stopping. I got some Lent lilies in Rouen, and have some celandines growing in moss, so it looks like spring in my bunk.

Thursday, March 11th.

Yesterday we took a long time getting to the ship from R., and unloaded at 10 p.m. Why we had no warning about the departure of the train (and so nearly got left behind) was because it was an emergency call suddenly to clear the hospitals at R. to make room for 600 more expected from the Front.

We are being rushed up again without being stopped at Rouen for the first time on record, so I suppose there is a good deal doing. (There was – at Neuve Chapelle.)

It is a comfort to remember that the men themselves don't grudge or question what happens to them, and the worse they're wounded the more they say, 'I think I'm lucky; my mate next me got killed.'

The birds are singing like anything now, and all the buds are coming out, and the banks and woods are a mass of primroses.

Friday, March 12th.

We came straight through Boulogne in the night, and have been stuck half way to the Front all day; I don't know why.

Saturday, March 13th.

We woke at the railhead for Béthune this morning, and cleared there and at the next place, mostly wounded and some Indians.

It was frightfully interesting up there to-day; we saw the famous German prisoners taken at Neuve Chapelle being entrained, and we could hear our great bombardment going on – the biggest ever known in any war. The feeling of Advance is in the air already, and even the wounded are exulting in it. The Indians have bucked up like anything. We are on our way down now, and shall probably unload at B.

No time for more now.

11 p.m. We unloaded at B. by 10 p.m., and are now on our way up again; shortest time we've ever waited – one hour after the last patient is off. A.T.'s have been tearing up empty and back full all day, and are all being unloaded at B., so that they can go quickly up again. B. has been emptied before this began.

They were an awfully brave lot of badly woundeds to-day, but they always are. Just now they don't mind anything – even getting hit by our artillery by mistake. Some of them who were near enough to see the effect of our bombardment on the enemy's trenches say they saw men, legs, and arms shot into the air. And the noise! – they gasp in telling you about it. 'You could never believe it,' they say. An officer told me exactly how many guns from 9.2's downwards we used, all firing at once. And poor fat Germans, and thin Germans, and big Germans, and little Germans at the other end of it.

A man of mine with his head shattered and his hand shot through was trephined last night, and his longitudinal sinus packed with gauze. He was on the train at 9 this morning, and actually improved during the day! He came to in the afternoon enough to remark, as if he were doing a French exercise, 'You-are-a-good-Nurse!' The next time he woke he said it again, and later on with great difficulty he gave me the address of his girl, to whom I am to write a post-card. I do hope they'll pull him through.

Sunday, March 14th, 4 p.m.
Just bringing down another load. I have a hundred and twenty wounded alone; the train is packed.

No time for more – the J.J.'s are swarming.

We unloaded at B. yesterday evening, and were off again within an hour or two.

Monday, March 15th, 2.30 a.m.
Woke up just as we arrived at Bailleul to hear most incessant cannonade going on I ever heard, even at Ypres. The sky is continually lit up with the flashes from the guns – it is a pitch-dark night – and you can hear the roar of the howitzers above the thud-thud of the others. I think we are too far N. for there to be any French 75's in it. I had to wake Sister D. to see it, as she had never seen anything like it before. We are only a few miles away from it.

Must try and sleep now, as we shall have a heavy day to-day, but it is no lullaby.

4.30 p.m. Just time for a scrawl. The train is packed with wounded, most of whom, including the poor sitting-ups, are now dead asleep from exhaustion. The British Army is fighting and marching all night now. The Clearing Hospitals get 800 in at a time, many with no dressings on. We have twenty-seven officers on this train alone.

I have a boy of 22 with both legs off. He is dazed and white, and wants shifting very often. Each time you fix him up he says, 'That's champion.'

Forty of them were shelled in their billets.

The Germans are said to be, some of them, fighting in civilian clothes till they get their uniforms. The men say there are hundreds of young boys and old men among them; they are making a desperate effort and bringing everything they've got into it now.

Later. We also have mumps, measles, scarlet fever, and diphtheria in the infectious coach.

A baby lieut. with measles showed me some marvellous sketch-maps of German trenches and positions he'd made from observations through a periscope. He also had the very latest thing in sectional war maps, numbered in squares, showing every tree, farm, and puddle and trench: a place with four cross-roads was called 'Confusion Corner', leading to a farm called 'Rest-and-be-Thankful'.

10 p.m. Just got them all off after a strenuous day, and we are to go up again at 11 p.m.

The two German divisions that reinforced are giving us a tremendous lot to do.

It is just as well that this department was prepared for this, as it all goes like clockwork and an enormous amount of suffering is saved by their preparedness.

The amount that cannot be saved is grim enough.

Must go to bed.

Tuesday, March 16th.
We loaded up very early this morning with 316 Indians, and are just getting into Boulogne. I expect we shall be sent up again this evening.

One of the Sikhs wailed before, during, and after his hand was dressed. A big Mussulman stuffed his hanky between his teeth and bit on it, and never uttered, and it was a much worse one. What was he to do with crying, he said; it was right for it to be done. May God bring blessings on my head; whereas it was full of pain, lo, now it was atcha.

Wednesday, March 17th.

I didn't tell you that yesterday a kind I.M.S. colonel at the place where we took the Indians on showed us a huge pile of used shell cases near the station, and we all had some. I've got a twelve-pounder and a sixteen-pounder, like my pom-poms, only huge. Next time he's going to get us some Gurkha's kukries. On the way down a little Gurkha happened to get off the train for a minute, and when he looked round the train had gone past him. He ran after it, and perched on one of the buffers till the next stop, when he reappeared, trembling with fright, but greeted with roars of amusement by the other Gurkhas.

We had some more to-day, including twelve with mumps, and one who insisted on coming with his mumpy friend though quite well himself!

We woke this morning at Merville, one of the railheads for Neuve Chapelle, and loaded up very early – guns going as hard as ever. Mine were a very bad lot – British (except the twelve native mumpers), including some brave Canadians. They kept me very busy till the moment of unloading, which is a difficult and painful business with these bad ones; but the orderlies are getting very gentle and clever with them. I had among them eight Germans, several mere boys. One insisted on kissing my hand, much to the orderlies' amusement.

(A truckful of pigs outside is making the most appalling noise. 11 p.m. I am writing in bed. We generally move up about 11.30 p.m.)

Every journey we hear thrilling accounts, rumours, and forecasts, most of which turn out to be true. We have had a lot of the St Eloi people.

There were several versions of a story of some women being found in a captured German trench. One version said they were French captives, another that they were German wives.

In one compartment were five Tommies being awfully kind to one German; and yet if he had a rifle, and they had theirs, he'd be a dead man.

The hospitals at Boulogne are so busy that no one goes off duty, and they are operating all night.

We had time for a blow across the bridge after unloading, and I happened to meet my friend S. (who was at Havre). She is on night duty, and they are grappling with those awful cases all night as hard as they can go. Four were taken out of the motor ambulances dead this week; the jolting is the last straw for the worst ones; it can't possibly be helped, 'but it seems a pity.'

In all this rush we happen to have had nights in bed, which makes all the difference.

The pigs still squeal, but I must try and go to sleep.

Thursday, March 18th.
We have had an off-day to-day at the place of woods and commons, which I hope and trust means that things are slackening off. It doesn't do to look ahead at what must be coming, now the ground is drying up before the job is finished; but we can be thankful for the spells of rest that come for the poor army.

We had a heavenly ramble this morning, and found blue periwinkles and anemones in the woods, but no primroses. Lots of palm and gorse. Robins, willow-wrens, and yellow-hammers were singing, the darlings, much prettier music than guns, and it is good to get away from the sound of motors and trains and whistles.

We also had home-made bread and butter to-day out of the village, which caused more excitement than the Russian successes. We are having much nicer food since the French chef left, and it costs us exactly half as much.

Friday, March 19th.
On the way down. Woke up at Bailleul, and loaded early wounded and sick. Not such severe cases among the wounded,

but several pneumonias, enterics, &c., besides measles, diphtheria, and scarlet.

Very cold windy day, with snow on the ground and showers of snow at intervals.

Some of mine are from the St Eloi, fighting last Sunday and Monday.

Some of N.'s regiment were badly caught between two ruined houses, each containing Maxims and machine-guns. They had just been reinforced by some young recruits of K.'s Army who detrained that night to go straight into the charge. 'They come on well, them youngsters,' said an old soldier, 'but they got terrible mowed down. We lost nine officers in a quarter of an hour.'

It has been a very costly splash altogether.

One officer on the train has fourteen wounds.

Saturday, March 20th, Boulogne.
The hospitals here have been pretty well emptied home now, and are ready for the next lot.

Here we have been standing by all day while a big Committee at Abbeville is settling whether our beloved and beautiful No.— A.T. is to be handed back to the French railway; and if so, whether it will be replaced by inferior French carriages, or whether one of the four new British trains that are coming will be handed over to us, or whether all the *personnel* will be disbanded and dispersed. I have a feeling that its day is over, but perhaps things will turn out better than that.

I have been for five walks to-day, including a bask in the sun on the sands, and a bath at the Club and a visit to the nice old R.C. church and the flower-market.

Tuesday, March 23rd, 9 p.m.
Waiting all day at G.H.Q.; things are unusually quiet; one train has been through with only ninety, and another with a hundred. We went for a walk along the canal this morning with the wee puppy, and this afternoon saw over the famous jute factory Convalescent Home, where they have a thousand beds under one roof: it is like a town divided into long wards, – dining-

rooms, recreation rooms, dressing station, chiropodist, tailor's shop, &c – by shoulder-high canvas or sailcloth screens; they have outside a kitchen, a boiler, a disinfector for clothes, and any amount of baths. They have a concert every Saturday night. The men looked so absolutely happy and contented with cooked instead of trench food, and baths and games and piano, and books and writing, &c. They stay usually ten days, and are by the tenth day supposed to be fit enough for the trenches again; it often saves them a permanent breakdown from general causes, and is a more economical way of treating small disablements than sending them to the Base Hospitals. Last week they had five hundred wounded to treat, and two of the M.O.'s had to take a supply-train of seven hundred slightly wounded down to Rouen with only two orderlies. They had a bad journey. I had a French class after tea. We are now expecting to-day's London papers, which are due here about 9 p.m.

Have got some Hindustani to learn for my next lesson (from Sister B.), so will stop this.

Wednesday, March 24th.
Moved on at 11 p.m. and woke up at Chocques; a few smallish guns going. Loaded up there very early and at two other places, and are now nearly back to Boulogne, mostly wounded and a few Indians; some of them are badly damaged by bombs.

The men in the Neuve Chapelle touch were awfully disappointed that they weren't allowed to push on to Lille. The older men say wonderful things of K.'s boys: 'The only fault we 'ave to find wi' 'em is that they expose theirselves too much. 'Keep your 'eads down!' we 'ave to say all the time. All they wants is to charge.'

According to the men, we shall be busy again at the end of this week.

Midnight. On way to coast near Havre where No.— G.H. is. Put all worst cases off at B., the rest mostly sleeping peacefully. Passed a place on coast not far S. of B., where six hundred British workmen are working from 7 a.m. to 10 p.m. building hospital huts for 12,000 beds, a huge encampment, ready for future business.

Have seen cowslips and violets on wayside. Lovely moonlight night. Train running very smoothly.

Thursday, March 25th.
There is a great deal of very neat and elaborate glass market-gardening going on round Rouen: it looks from the train an unbroken success; thousands of fat little plants with their glass hats off and thousands more with them on, and very little labour that can be seen. But the vegetables we buy for our mess are not particularly cheap.

9 p.m., *R.*— There are three trains waiting here, or rather at S., which means a blessed lull for the people in the firing line.

There was a day or two after Neuve Chapelle when the number of wounded overflowed the possibilities of 'collection'; the stretcher-bearers were all hit and the stretchers were all used, and there were not enough medical officers to cope with the numbers (extra ones were hurried up from the Base Hospitals very quickly), and if you wanted to live you had to walk or crawl, or stay behind and die. We had a Canadian on who told me last

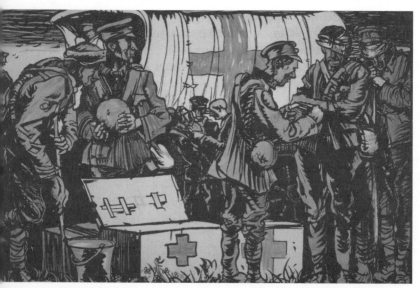

Red Cross poster showing the prevalence of Red Cross equipment.

night that he should never forget the stream of wounded dragging themselves along that road from Neuve Chapelle to Estaires who couldn't be found room for in the motor ambulances. Two trains picked them up there, and there were many deaths on the trains and in the motor ambulances. The 'Evacuation' was very thorough and rapid to the bases and to the ships, but in any great battle involving enormous casualties on both sides there must be some gaps you can't provide for.

Friday, March 26th.
At Sotteville all day.

Saturday, March 27th.
Ditto. Piercing cold winds and no heating for a month past.

Sunday, March 28th.
Ditto.
Monday, March 29th.
Ditto.

Tuesday, March 30th.
Ditto. This cold wind has dried up the mud everywhere, and until to-day there's been a bright sun with it.

The men clean the train and play football, and the M.O.'s take the puppy out, and everybody swears a great deal at a fate which no one can alter, and we are all craving for our week-old mails.

Wednesday, March 31st.
We actually acquired an engine and got a move on at 4 o'clock this morning, and are now well away north. Just got out where we stopped by a fascinating winding river, and got some brave marsh-marigolds.

5 p.m. – Just getting into Boulogne.

BILLETS: LIFE AT THE
BACK OF THE FRONT

April 2, 1915, to April 29, 1915.

Good Friday and Easter, 1915—The Maire's Château—A
walk to Beuvry—The new billet—The guns—A Taube—The
Back of the Front—A soldier's funeral—German Machine-
guns—Gas fumes—The Second Battle of Ypres.

Good Friday, April 2nd.
We got into Boulogne on Wednesday from Sotteville at 5 p.m.,
and as soon as the train pulled up a new Sister turned up
'to replace Sister ——', so I prepared for the worst and fully
expected to be sent to Havre or Étretat or Rouen, and began to
tackle my six and a half months' accumulation of belongings.
In the middle of this Miss —— from the Matron-in-Chief
arrived with my Movement Orders 'to proceed forthwith to
report to the O.C. of No.— Field Ambulance for duty', so hell
became heaven, and here I am at railhead waiting for a motor
ambulance to take me and my baggage to No.— F.A. wherever
it is to be found.

The Railway Transport Officer at Boulogne let me come up
as far as St Omer (or rather the next waiting place beyond),
on No.— A.T., and get sent on by the R.T.O. there. We waited

there all yesterday, lovely sunny day, and in the evening the R.T.O. sent me on in a supply train which was going to the railhead for No.— F.A. The officer in charge of it was very kind, and turned out of his carriage for me into his servant's, and apologised for not having cleared out every scrap of his belongings. The Mess of No.— saw me off, with many farewell jokes and witticisms.

This supply train brings up one day's rations to the 1st Corps from Havre, and takes a week to do it there and back. This happens daily for one corps alone, so you can imagine the work of the A.S.C. at Havre. At railhead he is no longer responsible for his stuff when the lorries arrive and take up their positions end on with the trucks. They unload and check it, and it is done in four hours. That part of it is now going on.

When we got to railhead at 10.15 p.m. the R.T.O. said it was too late to communicate with the Field Ambulance, and so I slept peacefully in the officer's bunk with my own rugs and cushion. We had tea about 9 p.m. I had had dinner on No.—.

This morning the first thing I saw was No.— A.T. slumbering in the sun on the opposite line, so I might just as well have come up in her, except that there was another Sister in my bed.

After a sketchy wash in the supply train, and a cup of early tea from the officer's servant, I packed up and went across to No.— for breakfast; many jeers at my having got the sack so soon.

The R.T.O. has just been along to say that Major —— of No.— Clearing Hospital here will send me along in one of his motor ambulances.

11 a.m. Had an interesting drive here in the M.A. through a village packed with men billeted in barns and empty houses – the usual aeroplane buzzing overhead, and a large motor ambulance convoy by the wayside.

We are in the town itself, and the building is labelled No.— F.A. Dressing Station for Officers. The men are in a French Civil Hospital run very well by French nuns, and it has been decided to keep the French and English nurses quite separate, so the only difference between the two hospitals is that the one for the men has French Sisters, with R.A.M.C. orderlies and M.O.'s, and the other for officers has English Sisters, with R.A.M.C. orderlies and M.O.'s. There are forty-seven beds here (all officers). One Army Sister in charge, myself next, and two staff nurses – one on night duty. There are two floors; I shall have charge of the top floor.

We are billeted out, but I believe mess in the hospital.

All this belongs to the French Red Cross, and is lent to us.

The surgical outfit is much more primitive even than on the train, as F.A.'s may carry so little. The operating theatre is at the other hospital.

As far as I can see at present we don't have the worst cases here, except in a rush like Neuve Chapelle.

It will be funny to sleep in a comfortable French bed in an ordinary bedroom again. It will be rather like Le Mans over again, with a billet to live in, and officers to look after, but I shall miss the Jocks and the others.

Later. Generals and 'Red Hats' simply bristle around. A collection of them has just been in visiting the sick officers. We had a big Good Friday service at 11, and there is another at 6 p.m. The Bishop of London is coming round to-day.

Still Good Friday, 10 p.m. Who said Active Service? I am writing this in a wonderful mahogany bed, with a red satin quilt, in a panelled room, with the sort of furniture drawing-rooms have on the stage, and electric light, and medallions and bronzes, and oil-paintings and old engravings, and blue china and mirrors all about. It is a huge house like a Château, on the Place, where Generals and officers are usually billeted. The fat and smiling caretaker says she's had two hundred since the war. She insisted on pouring eau-de-Cologne into my hot bath. It is really a lovely house, with polished floors and huge tapestry pictures up the staircase. And all this well within range of the German guns. After last night, in the A.S.C officer's kind but musty little chilly second-class carriage, it is somewhat of a change. And I hadn't had my clothes off for three days and two nights. This billet is only for one night; to-morrow I expect I shall be in some grubby little room near by. It has taken the Town Commandant, the O.C. of

No.— F.A., a French interpreter, and an R.H.A. officer and several N.C.O.'s and orderlies, to find me a billet – the town is already packed tight, and they have to continue the search to-morrow.

This afternoon I went all over the big French hospital where our men are. The French nuns were charming, and it was all very nice. The women's ward is full of women and girls *blessées* by shells, some with a leg off and fractured – all very cheerful.

One shell the other day killed thirty-one and wounded twenty-seven – all Indians.

I am not to start work till to-morrow, as the wards are very light; nearly all the officers up part of the day, so at 6 p.m. I went to the Bishop of London's mission service in the theatre. A staff officer on the steps told me to go to the left of the front row (where all the red hats and gold hats sit), but I funked that and sat modestly in the last row of officers. There were about a hundred officers there, and a huge solid pack of men; no other woman at all. The Bishop, looking very white and tired but very happy, took the service on the stage, where a Padre was thumping the hymns on the harmonium (which shuts up into a sort of matchbox). It was a voluntary service, and you know the nearer they are to the firing line the more they go to church. It was extraordinarily moving. The Padre read a sort of liturgy for the war taken from the Russians, far finer than any of ours; we had printed papers, and the response was 'Lord, have mercy', or 'Grant this, O Lord'. It came each time like bass clockwork.

Troops are just marching by in the dark. Hundreds passed the hospital this afternoon. I must go to sleep.

The Bishop dashed in to see our sick officers here, and then motored off to dine with the Quartermaster-General. He's had great services with the cavalry and every other brigade.

Easter Eve, 10 p.m.
Have been on duty all day till 5 p.m. They are nearly all 'evacuated' in a few days, so you are always getting a fresh lot in.

Another Army Sister turned up to-day in a motor from Poperinghe to take the place of the two who were originally here, who have now gone.

At six this morning big guns were doing their Morning Hate very close to us, but they have been quiet all day. Two days ago the village two and a half miles south-east of us was shelled.

I found my own new billet this morning before going on duty; it is in a very old little house over a shop in a street off the big Place. It is a sort of attic, and I am not dead sure whether it is clean on top and lively underneath, but time will show. The shop lady and her daughter Maria Thérèse are full of zeal and kindness to make me comfortable, but they stayed two hours watching me unpack and making themselves agreeable! And when I came in from dinner from the café, where we now have our meals (quite decent), she and papa and M.T. drew up a chair for me to *causer* in their parlour, to my horror.

At 8 p.m. the town suddenly goes out like a candle; all lights are put out and the street suddenly empty. After that, at intervals, only motorcyclists buzz through and regiments tramp past going back to billets. They sound more warlike than anything. Such a lot are going by now.

Easter Sunday.

3 p.m. The service at 7 this morning in the theatre was rather wonderful. Rows of officers and packs of men.

We have been busy in the ward all the morning. I'm off 2-5, and shall soon go out and take E.'s chocolate Easter eggs to the men in the hospice. The officers have any amount of cigarettes, chocs., novels, and newspapers.

A woman came and wept this morning with my billeter over their two sons, who are prisoners, not receiving the parcels of *tabac* and *pain* and *gateaux* that they send. They think we ought to starve the German prisoners to death!

This morning in the ward I suddenly found it full of Gold Hats and Red Tabs; three Generals and their A.D.C.'s visiting the sick officers.

Easter Monday.

It is a pouring wet day, and the mud is Flanderish. Never was there such mud anywhere else. A gunner-major has just been telling me you get a fine view of the German positions from the Cathedral tower here, and can see shells bursting like the pictures in 'The Sphere'. He said his guns had the job of peppering La Bassée the last time they shelled this place, and they gave it such a dusting that this place has been let severely alone since. He thinks they'll have another go at this when we begin to get hold of La Bassée, but the latter is a very strong position. It begins to be 'unhealthy' to get into any of the villages about three miles from here, which are all heaps of bricks now.

I'm leaving my billet to-morrow, as they want us to be in one house. And our house is the Maire's Château, the palatial one, so we shall live in the lap of luxury as never before in this country! And have hot baths with eau-de-Cologne every night, or cold every morning. And the woman is going to *faire* our cuisine there for us, so we shan't have to wait hours in the café for our meals. There is only one waiter at the café, who is a beautiful, composed, wrapt, silent girl of 16, who will soon be dead of overwork. She is not merely pretty, but beautiful, with the manners of a princess!

I shall be glad to get away from my too kind billeters; every night I have to sit and *causer* before going to bed, and Ma-billeter watches me in and out of bed, and tells me my nightgown is *très pratique*, and just like the officers Anglais have. But she calls me with a lovely cup of coffee in the morning. They've been so kind that I dread telling them I've got to go.

An officer was brought in during the night with a compound-fractured arm. He stuck a very painful dressing like a brick to-day, and said to me afterwards, 'I've got three kids at home; they'll be awfully bucked over this!' He had said it was 'nothing to write home about'.

Another, who is chaffing everybody all day long, was awfully impressed because a man in his company – I mean platoon – who had half his leg blown off, said when they came to pick him up, 'Never mind me – take so-and-so first' – 'just like those chaps you read of in books, you know.' It was decided that he meant Sir Philip Sidney.

Yesterday afternoon I had a lovely time taking round chocolate Easter eggs to our wounded in the French hospital. The sweetest, merriest *Ma-Sœur* took me round, and insisted on all the orderlies having one too. They adore her, and stand up and salute when she comes into the ward; and we had enough for the *jeunes filles* and the grannies in the women's ward of *blessées*. They were a huge success. Those men get very few treats. She also showed me the Maternity Ward.

Tuesday, April 6th, 10 p.m.

I am writing in bed in my lovely little room overlooking the garden, and facing some nice red roofs and both the old Towers of the town (one dating from *le temps des Espagnols*) in *le Château*, instead of in my attic in the narrow street where you heard the tramp of the men who *viennent des tranches* in the night. We had a lovely dinner, served by the fat and *très aimable* Marie in a small, panelled dining-room, with old oak chairs and real silver spoons (the first I've met since August). So don't waste any pity for the hardships of War! And an officer with a temperature of 103° explained that he'd been sleeping for sixteen days on damp sandbags 'among the dead Germans'.

Nothing coming in anywhere, but when it does begin we shall get them.

The A.D.M.S. is going to arrange for us to go up with one of his motor ambulances to one of the advance dressing stations where the first communication trench begins! It is at the corner of a road called 'Harley Street', which he says is 'too unhealthy', where I mayn't be taken. Won't it be thrilling to see it all?

Officers' 'trench talk' is exactly like the men's, only in a different language.

It has been wet and windy again, so I did not explore when I was off this afternoon, but did my unpacking and settling in here. With so many moves I have got my belongings into a high state of mobilisation, and it doesn't take long.

Last night at the café, one of the despatch riders played Chopin, Tchaikowsky, and Elgar like a professional. It was jolly. The officers are awfully nice to do with on the whole.

Wednesday, April 7th. In bed, 10.30 p.m.

It has been a lovely day after last night's and yesterday's heavy rain. We are busy all day admitting and evacuating officers. The lung one had to be got ready in a hurry this morning, and Mr L. took him down specially to the train.

A very nice Brigade-Major came in, in the night, with a shell wound in the shoulder. This morning a great jagged piece was dug out, with only a local anæsthetic, and he stuck it like a brick, humming a tune when it became unbearable and gripping on to my hand.

I was off at 5 p.m., and went to dig out Marie Thérèse from my old billet, to come with me to Beuvry, the village about two and a half miles away that was shelled last week; it is about half-way to the trenches from here. It was a lovely sunsetty evening, and there was a huge stretch of view, but it was not clear enough to make anything out of the German line. She has a tante and a grandmère there, and has a '*laisser-passer soigner une tante malade*' which she has to show to the sentry at the bridge. I get through without. The tante is not at all *malade* – she is a cheery old lady who met us on the road. M.T. pointed me out all the shell holes. We met and passed an unending stream of khaki, the men marching back from their four days in the trenches, infant officers and all steadily trudging on with the same coating of mud from head to foot, packs and rifles carried anyhow, and the Trench Look, which can never be described, and which is grim to the last degree. Each lot had a tail of limping stragglers in ones and twos and threes. I talked to some of these, and they said they'd had a very 'rough' night last night – pouring rain – water up to their knees, and standing to all night expecting an attack which didn't come off; but some mines had been exploded meant for their trench, but luckily they were ten yards out in their calculations, and they only got smothered instead of blown to bits. And they were sticking all this while we were snoring in our horrible, warm, soft beds only a few miles away. We went on past some of the famous brick stacks through the funny little village full of billets to the church, where *le Salut* was going on. We passed a dressing station of No.— Field Ambulance. The grandmère had two sergeants billeted with her who seemed pleased to have a friendly chat. Some of the men I said good-night to were so surprised (not knowing our grey coat and hat), I heard them say to each other 'English!' Marie Thérèse simply adores the *Anglais* – they are so *gais*, such *bon courage*, they laugh always and sing – and they have '*beaucoup de fiancées françaises pour passer le temps*'! She told me they had yesterday a boy of eighteen who was always *triste*, but *bien poli*, and he knows six languages and comes from the University of London. When he left for the trenches he said, '*Je vais à la mort*,' but he has promised to come and see them on Saturday or Sunday, '*s'il n'est pas mort, ou blessé*,' she said, as an afterthought. Her own young man is *à la Guerre*, and she is making her trousseau. They do beautiful embroidery on linen.

I was pretty tired when we got back at 8 o'clock, as it was a good five-mile walk, part of the way on fiendish cobble-stones, and we are on our feet all day at the Dressing Station. But I am very fit, and all the better for the excellent fresh food we have here. No more tins of anything, thank goodness!

Thursday, April 8th.
Talking of billets, a General and his Staff are coming to this Château to-morrow and we three have got to turn out, possibly to a house opposite on the same square, which is empty. We live in terror of unknown Powers-that-Be suddenly sending us down. The C.O. and everyone here are very keen that we should be as comfortably billeted as possible. He said to-day, 'Later on you may get an awful place to live in.' Of course we are aiming at becoming quite indispensable! If you can once get your Medical Officers to depend on you for having everything they want at hand, and for making the patients happy and contented, and the orderlies in good order, they soon get to think they can't do without you.

There are two nice tea-shops where all the officers of the 1st and 2nd Divisions go and have tea.

On Saturday morning they sent three hundred shells into Cuinchy, in revenge for their trench blown up (see to-day's *Communiqué* from Sir J.F.).

Friday, April 9th, 10.30 p.m.

An empty house was found for us on the same square, left exactly as it was when the owners left when the place was shelled. It was filthy from top to toe, but we have found a girl called Gabrielle to be our servant, and she has made a good start in the cleaning to-day. There are three bedrooms – mine is a funny little one built out at the back, down three steps, with two windows overlooking a corner of the square and our road past the hospital.

It is my fourth billet here in a week, and Gabrielle and I have made it quite habitable by collecting things from other parts of the house. We are back in our own rugs and blankets again without sheets, and there is no water on yet, but we filled our hot-water bottles at the hospital, and are quite warm and cosy, and locked up – I shall have to let Gabrielle in at 6.30 to-morrow morning. She is going to shop and cook for us, with help from the kind Marie at the Château, who is aghast at our present more military mode of living. The Château is now swarming with Staff Officers, to whom Marie pays far less attention than she does to us!

When the wind is in the right direction you can hear the rifle firing as well as the guns – and they are often shelling aeroplanes on a fine day. We have two bad cases in to-night – one wounded in the lung, and one medical transferred from downstairs, where the slight medicals are.

A Captain of the ——, hit in the back this morning when he was crossing in the open to visit a post in his trench, has a little freckled Jock for his servant, who dashed out to bring him in when he fell. 'Most gallant, you know,' he said. They adore each other. Jock stands to attention, salutes, and says 'Yes'm' when I gave him an order. Their friends troop in to see them as soon as they hear they're hit. So many seem to have been wounded before – nearly all, in fact.

Letters are coming in very irregularly, I don't quite know why.

Saturday, April 10th, 10.30 p.m.

It is difficult to settle down to sleep to-night: the sky is lit up with flashes and star-shells, and every now and then a big bang shakes the house, above the almost continuous thud, thudding, and the barking of the machine-guns and the crackling of rifle firing; they are bringing in more to-day, both here and at the Hospice, and we are tired enough to go to sleep as if we were at home; I shouldn't wonder if the Night Sister had a busy night.

We had to rig up our day-room for an operation this evening – they have always taken them over to the Hospice, where they have a very swanky modern theatre.

We couldn't manage to get any food to-day for Gabrielle to cook for us, as our rations hadn't come up, so we went back to the café. She has been busy nettoying all day, and the house feels much cleaner.

The dead silence, darkness, and emptiness of the streets after 8 o'clock are very striking.

Sunday, April 11th.

This afternoon they shelled Beuvry (the village I went to with Marie Thérèse on Wednesday) and wounded eleven women and children; the advanced dressing station of No.— F.A. took them in. The promise to send us in one of the M.A.'s to 'Harley Street' (the name of the first communication trench) has been taken back until things quiet down a little. There was an air battle just above us this evening – a Taube sailing serenely along not very high, and not altering her course or going up one foot, for all the shells that promptly peppered the sky all round her. You hear a particular kind of bang and then gaze at the Taube; suddenly a shining ball of white smoke appears close to her, and uncurls itself in the sun against the blue of the sky. As it begins to uncurl you hear the explosion, and however much you admire the German's pluck, and hope he'll dodge them safely, you can't help hoping also that the next one will get him and that he'll come crashing down. Isn't it beastly? It was so near that the French were calling out excitedly, '*Touché! Il descend*,' but he got away all right.

Another officer dangerously wounded was transferred to my ward to-day from the French hospital. He was feebly grappling with a Sevenpenny which he could neither hold nor read. 'Anything to take my thoughts off that beastly war!' he said.

A small parcel of socks, cigs., and chocs, came to-day. Soon after, I found the road below was covered with exhausted trench stragglers resting on the kerb, the very men for the parcel. They had all that and one mouth-organ – wasn't it lucky? One Jock said, 'That's the first time I've heard a woman speak English since I left Southampton six months ago!'

Gabrielle cooked a very nice supper for us to-night – which I dished up when we came in. It is much more fun camping out in our own little empty house than in the grand Château – but I didn't have time to look at nearly all the lovely engravings there.

Streams of columns have been passing all day; one gun-team had to turn back because one of the off horses jibbed and refused to go any farther.

Though it is past 11 p.m. the sounds outside are too interesting to go to sleep; the bangs are getting louder; those who *viennent des tranches* are tramping down and transport waggons rattling up!

Monday, April 12th.
No mail to-day. This has been a very quiet day, fewer columns, aeroplanes, and guns, and the three bad officers holding their own so far. The others come and go.

Tuesday, April 13th.
There is something quite fiendish about the crackling of the rifle firing to-night, and every now and then a gun like 'Mother' speaks and shakes the town. Last night it was quite quiet. All leave has been stopped to-day, and there are the wildest rumours going about of a big naval engagement, the forcing of the Narrows, and the surrender of St Mihiel, and anything else you like!

These Medical Officers have always hung on to the most hopeless, both here and at the Hospice, beyond the last hope, and when they pull through there is great rejoicing.

It doesn't seem somehow the right thing to do, to undress and get into bed with these crashes going on, but I suppose staying up won't stop it!

Wednesday, April 14th.

Very quiet day; it always is after exciting rumours which come to nothing! But it has been noisier than usual in the daytime. I rested in my off-time and didn't go out.

The Victoria League sent some awfully nice lavender bags to-day, and some tins of Keating's, which will be of future use, I expect. Just now, one is mercifully and strangely free from the Minor Scourges of War.

The German trenches captured at Neuve Chapelle, and now occupied by us, are full of legs and arms, which emerge when you dig. Some are still caught on the barbed wire and can't be taken away.

We are not being at all clever with our rations just now, and manage to have indescribably nasty and uneatable meals! But we shall get it better in time, by taking a little more trouble over it.

We had scrambled eggs to-night, which I made standing on a chair, because the gas-ring is so high, and Sister holding up a very small dim oil-lamp. But they were a great success. And then we had soup with fried potatoes in it! and tea.

Thursday, April 15th.

This afternoon has been a day to remember. We've had our journey up to the firing line, to a dressing station just over half a mile from the first line of German trenches! It is between the two villages of Givenchy and Cuinchy, this side of La Bassée. The journey there was through the village I walked to with Marie Thérèse (which has been shelled twice since we came), and along the long, wide, straight road the British Army now knows so well – paved in the middle and a straight line of poplars on each side. As far as you could see it was covered with two streams of khaki, with an occasional string of French cavalry – one stream going up to the trenches after their so many days' 'rest', and the other coming from the trenches to their 'rest'. We soon got up to some old German trenches from which we drove them months ago; they run parallel with the road. On the other side we saw one of our own Field Batteries, hidden in the scrub of a hedge – not talking at the moment. There were also some French batteries hidden behind an embankment. 'The German guns are trained always on this road,' said our A.S.C. driver cheerfully, 'but they don't generally begin not till about 4 o'clock,' so, as it was then 2.30, we weren't alarmed. They know it is used for transport and troops and often send a few shells on to it. We sat next him and he did showman. Before long we got into the area of ruined houses – and they are a sight! They spell War, and War only – nothing else (but perhaps an earthquake?) could make such awful desolation; in a few of the smaller cottages with a roof on, the families had gone back to live in a sort of patched-up squalor, but all the bigger houses and parts of streets were mere jagged shells. The two villages converge just where we turned a corner from the La Bassée road into a lane on our left where the dressing station is. A little farther on is 'Windy Corner', which is 'a very hot place'. We had before this passed some of our own reserve unoccupied trenches, some with sandbags for parapets, but now we suddenly found ourselves with a funny barricade of different coloured and shaped doors, taken from the ruined houses, about 8 feet high on our right. This was to prevent the German snipers from seeing our transport or M.A.'s pass down that lane to the communication trench, which has its beginning at the ruined house which is used by the F.A. as one of its advanced dressing stations. It is called No. 1 Harley Street. Here we got out, and the first person we saw was Sergt. P., who was theatre orderly in No. 7 at Pretoria. He greeted us warmly and took us to Capt. R., who was the officer in charge. He also was most awfully kind and showed us all over his place. We went first into his two cellars, where the wounded are taken to be dressed, instead of above, where they might be shelled. They had a queer collection of furniture – a table for dressings, and some oddments of chairs, including two carved oak dining-room chairs. Round the front steps is a barricade of sandbags against snipers' bullets. The officer's room above the cellars was quite nice and tidy, furnished from the ruined houses, and with a vase of daffodils! He had been told the day before to allow no one up the staircase, because snipers were on the look-out for the top windows, and if it were seen to be used as an observing station it might draw the shells. However, just before we left he changed his mind and took us up and showed us all the landmarks, including the famous brick-stacks, where there must be many German graves, but we all had to be very careful not to show ourselves. The garden at the back has a row of graves with flowers growing on them, and neat wooden crosses with little engraved tin plates on, with the name and regiment. One was, 'An unknown British Soldier'. There were no wounded in the D.S. this afternoon.

The orderlies showed us lots of interesting bits of German shells and time fuses, &c. The house was full of big holes, with dirty smart curtains, and hats and mirrors lying about the floors upstairs among the brickwork and ruins.

They then took us a little way down the communication trench called 'Hertford Street', under the 'Marble Arch' to 'Oxford Circus'! It is quite dry mud over bricks and very narrow, and goes higher than your head on the enemy side, and has zigzags very often. You can only go single file, and we had to wait in a zigzag to let a lot of men go by – they stream past almost continually. One officer invited us to come and see his dug-out, but it was farther along than we might go without being awfully in the way. We had before this given one stream of ingoing men all the cigarettes, chocolates, writing-paper, mouth-organs, Keating's, pencils, and newspapers we could lay hands on before we started, and we could have done with thousands of each. Every few minutes one of our guns talked with a startlingly loud noise somewhere near, but Captain R. said it was an exceptionally quiet day, and we didn't hear a single German gun or see any bursting shells. It was a particularly warm sunny day, and the men going into the trenches were so cheerful and jolly that it didn't seem at all tragic or depressing, and there was nothing but one's recollections of the Aisne and Ypres after what they call 'a show' to remind one what it all meant and what it might at any moment turn into. One hasn't had before the opportunities of seeing the men who are in it (and not at the Bases or on the Lines of Communication) while they are fit, but only after they are wounded or sick, and the contrast is very striking. All these after their 'rest' look fit and sunburnt and natural, and the one expression that never or rarely fails, whether fit, wounded, or sick, is the expression of acquiescence and going through with it that they all have. If it failed at all it was with the men with frost-bite and trench feet, who stuck it so long when winter first came on before they got the braziers, and in the long rains when they stood in mud and water to their waists. Now, thank Heaven, the ground is hard again.

I saw three small children playing about just behind the dressing station, where some men unloading a lorry were killed a few days ago. The women and children are all along the road, absolutely regardless of danger as long as they are allowed to stay in their own homes. The babies sit close up against the Tommies who are resting by the roadside.

We saw a great many wire entanglements, so thick that they look like a field of lavender a little way off. From the top windows of the ruined house we could see long lines of heads, picks and shovels, going single file down 'Hertford Street', but they couldn't be seen from the enemy side because of the parapet.

Friday, April 16th.
At about 7.30 this evening I was writing the day report when the sergeant came in with three candles and said an order had come for all lights to be put out and only candles used. So I had to put out all the lights and give the astonished officers my three candles between them, while the sergeant went out to get some more. The town looks very weird with all the street lamps out and only glimmers from the windows. It was kept pretty darkened before. It may be because of the Zeppelin at Bailleul on Wednesday, or another may be reported somewhere about.

This afternoon I saw a soldier's funeral, which I have never seen before. He was shot in the head yesterday, and makes the four hundred and eleventh British soldier buried in this cemetery. I happened to be there looking at the graves, and the French gravedigger told me there was to be another buried this afternoon. The gravedigger's wife and children are with the Allemands, he told me, the other side of La Bassée, and he has no news of them or they of him.

It was very impressive and moving, the Union Jack on the coffin (a thin wooden box) on the waggon, and a firing party, and about a hundred men and three officers and the Padre. It was a clear blue sky and sunny afternoon, and the Padre read beautifully and the men listened intently. The graves are dug trenchwise, very close together, practically all in one continuous grave, each with a marked cross. There is a long row of officers, and also seven Germans and five Indians.

The two Zeppelins reported last night must have gone to bed after putting out all our lights, as nothing happened anywhere.

The birds and buds in the garden opposite make one long for one's lost leave, but I suppose they will keep.

We have only nine officers in to-day; everything is very quiet everywhere, but troop trains are very busy.

10.30 p.m. It is getting noisy again. Some batteries on our right next the French lines are doing some thundering, and there are more star-shells than usual lighting up the sky on the left. They look like fireworks. They are sent up *in* the firing line to see if any groups of enemy are crawling up to our trenches in the dark. When they stop sending theirs up we have to get busy with ours to see what they're up to. It's funny to see that every night from your bedroom windows. They give a tremendous light as soon as they burst.

When I went into the big church for benediction this evening at 6.30, every estaminet and café and tea-shop was packed with soldiers, and also as usual every street and square. At seven o'clock they were all emptying, as there is an order to-day to close all cafés, &c., at seven instead of eight.

All lights are out again to-night.

Another aeroplane was being shelled here this evening.

Sunday, April 18th, 9.30 p.m.

It has been another dazzling day. A major of one of the Indian regiments came in this evening. He said the Boches are throwing stones across to our men wrapped in paper with messages like this written on them, 'Why don't you stop the War? We want to get home to our wives these beautiful days, and so do you, so why do you go on fighting?' The sudden beauty of the spring and the sun has made it all glaringly incongruous, and everyone feels it.

One badly wounded officer got it going out of his dug-out to attend to a man of his company who was hit by a sniper in an exposed place, one of his subalterns told me. His own account, of course, was a rambling story leaving that part entirely out.

This next shows how the Germans had left nothing to chance. They have about twelve machine-guns to every battalion, and are said to have had 12,000 when the War began. Passing through villages they pack ten of them into an innocent-looking cart with a false bottom. We captured some of these empty carts, and some time afterwards found them full of machine-guns!

Gold hats and red hats have been dropping in all day. They do on Sundays especially after Church Parade.

Saturday, April 24th.

We were watching hundreds of men pass by to-day, whistling and singing, on their way to the trenches.

News came to us this morning of the Germans having broken through the trench lines north of Ypres and shelled Poperinghe, which was out of range up to now, but it is not official.

The guns are very loud to-night; I hope they're keeping the Germans busy; something is sure to be done to draw them off the Ypres line.

Sunday, April 25th.

The plum-pudding was 'something to write home about!' and the Quartermaster sent us a tin of honey to-day, the first I've seen for nine months.

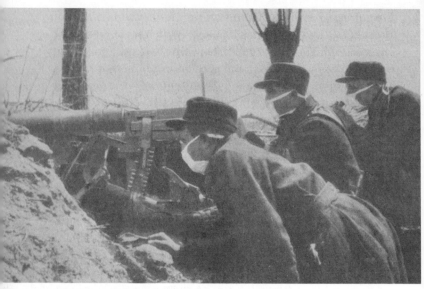

Troops wearing early rudimentary gas masks.

A General came round this morning. He said the Canadians and another regiment had given the Germans what for for this gas-fumes business north of Ypres, got the ground back and recovered the four guns. The beasts of Germans laid out a whole trench full of Zouaves with chlorine gas (which besides being poisonous is one of the most loathsome smells). Of course everyone is busy finding out how we can go one better now. But this afternoon the medical staffs of both these divisions have been trying experiments in a barn with chlorine gas, with and without different kinds of masks soaked with some antidote, such as lime. All were busy coughing and choking when they found the A.D.M.S. of the —— Division getting blue and suffocated; he'd had too much chlorine, and was brought here, looking very bad, and for an hour we had to give him fumes of ammonia till he could breathe properly. He will probably have bronchitis. But they've found out what they wanted to know – that you can go to the assistance of men overpowered by the gas, if you put on this mask, with less chance of finding yourself dead too when you got there. They don't lose much time finding these things out, do they?

On Saturday I shall be going on night duty for a month.

Monday, April 26th, 11 p.m.
We have been admitting, cutting the clothes off, dressing, and evacuating a good many to-day, and I think they are still coming in.

There is a great noise going on to-night, snapping and popping, and crackling of rifle firing and machine-guns, with the sudden roar of our 9.2's every few minutes. The thundery roll after them is made by the big shell bounding along on its way.

Two officers were brought in last night from a sap where they were overpowered by carbon monoxide. Three of them and a sergeant crawled along it to get out the bodies of another officer and a sergeant who'd been killed there by an explosion the day before; it leads into a crater in the German lines, and reaches under the German trenches, which we intended to blow up. But they were greeted by this poisonous gas last night, and the officer in front of these two suddenly became inanimate; each tried to pull the one in front out by the legs, but all became unconscious in turn, and only these two survived and were hauled out up twenty feet of rope-ladder. They will get all right.

The wounded ones are generally in 'the excited stage' when they arrive – some surprised and resentful, some relieved that it is no worse, and some very quiet and collapsed.

Captain —— showed me his periscope to-day; you bob down and look into it about level with his mattress, and then you see a picture of the garden across the road. He has seen one made by Ross with a magnifying lens in it so good that you can see the moustaches of the Boches in it from the bottom of your trench. The noise is getting so beastly I must knock off and read *Punch*.

Tuesday, April 27th.
Have been busy all day, and so have the guns. When the 15-inch howitzers began to talk the old concierge lady at the

O.D.S. trotted out to see *l'orage*, and found a cloudless sky, and, *mon Dieu*, it was *les canons*. It is a stupendous noise, like some gigantic angry lion. The official accounts of the second dash for Calais reach us through *The Times* two days after the things have happened, but the actual happenings filter along the line from St Omer (G.H.Q.) as soon as they happen, so we know there's been no real 'breaking through' that hasn't been made good, or partially made good, because if there had, the dispositions all along the line would have had to be altered, and that has not happened.

The ambulance trains are collecting the Ypres casualties straight from the convoys at Poperinghe, as we did at Ypres in October and November, and not through the Clearing Hospitals, which I believe have had to move farther back.

Wednesday, April 28th.
Here everything is as it has been for the last few days (except the weather, which is suddenly hot as summer), rather more casualties, but no rush, and the same crescendo of heavy guns. Some shells were dropped in a field just outside the town at 8.30 yesterday evening but did no damage.

Thursday, April 29th, 4 p.m.
The weather and the evenings are indescribably incongruous. Tea in the garden at home, deck-chairs, and Sweep under the walnut-tree come into one's mind, and before one's eyes and ears are motor ambulances and stretchers and dressings, and the everlasting noise of marching feet, clattering hoofs, lorries, and guns, and sometimes the skirl of the pipes. One day there was a real band, and everyone glowed and thrilled with the sound of it.

I strayed into a concert at 5.30 this evening, given by the Glasgow Highlanders to a packed houseful of men and officers. I took good care to be shown into a solitary box next the stage, as I was alone and guessed that some of the items would not be intended for polite female ears. The level of the talent was a high one, some good part songs, and two real singers, and some quite funny and clever comic; but one or two things made me glad of the shelter of my box. The choruses were fine. The last thing was a brilliant effort of the four part singers dressed as comic sailors, which simply made the house rock. Then suddenly, while they were still yelling, the first chords of the 'King' were played, and all the hundreds stood to attention in a pin-drop silence while it was played – not sung – much more impressive than the singing of it, I thought.

We have had some bad cases in to-day, and the boy with the lung is not doing so well.

My second inoculation passed off very quickly, and I have not been off duty for it.

FESTUBERT, MAY 9 AND MAY 16

May 6, 1915, to May 26, 1915.

The noise of war—Preparation—Sunday, May 9—The
barge—The officers' dressing station—Charge of the Black
Watch, May 9—Festubert, May 16—The French Hospital—
A bad night—Shelled out—Back at a Clearing Hospital—
'For duty at a Base Hospital.'

Thursday, May 6th, 3 a.m.
It was a very noisy day, and I didn't sleep after 2 p.m. There is
a good lot of firing going on to-night.

A very muddy officer of 6 ft. 4 was brought in early yesterday
morning with a broken leg, and it is a hard job to get him
comfortable in these short beds.

Yesterday at 4 a.m.I couldn't resist invading the garden
opposite which is the R.A. Headquarters. It is full of lovely
trees and flowers and birds. I found a blackbird's nest with
one egg in. From the upper windows of this place it makes
a perfect picture, with the peculiarly beautiful tower of the
Cathedral as a background.

Friday, May 7th, 1 a.m.
The noise is worse than anywhere in London, even the King's
Road. The din that a column of horse-drawn, bolt-rattling

waggons make over cobbles is literally deafening; you can't hear each other speak. And the big motor-lorries taking the 'munitions of war' up are almost as bad. These processions alternate with marching troops, clattering horses, and French engines all day, and very often all night, and in the middle of it all there are the guns. Tonight the rifle firing is crackling.

Sir John French and Sir Douglas Haig have been up here to-day, and everyone is telling everyone else when the great Attack is going to begin.

There are three field ambulances up here, and only work for two (—th and —th), so the —th is established in a huge school for 500 boys, where it runs a great laundry and bathing establishment. A thousand men a day come in for bath, disinfection, and clean clothes; 100 French women do the laundry work in huge tubs, and there are big disinfectors and drying and ironing rooms. The men of the F.A. do the sorting and all the work except the washing and ironing. And the beautifully-cared-for English cart-horses that belong to the F.A., and the waggons and the motor ambulances and the equipment, are all kept ready to move at a moment's notice.

Colonel —— showed me all over it this evening. It is done at a cost to the Government of 7d. per man, washed and clothed.

My blackbird has laid another egg.

Friday, May 7th, 10 p.m.
A pitch-dark night, raining a little, and only one topic – the Attack to-morrow morning.

The first R.A.M.C. barge has come up, and is lying in the canal ready to take on the cases of wounds of lung and abdomen, to save the jolting of road and railway; it is to have two Sisters, but I haven't seen them yet: shall go in the morning: went round this morning to see, but the barge hadn't arrived.

There are a few sick officers downstairs who are finding it hard to stick in their beds, with their regiments in this job close by. There is a house close by which I saw this morning with a dirty little red flag with a black cross on it, where the C.-in-C. and thirty commanders of the 1st Army met yesterday.

The news to-day of Hill 60 and the gases is another spur to the grim resolve to break through here, that can be felt and seen and heard in every detail of every arm. 'Grandmother' is lovingly talked about.

The town, the roads, and the canal banks this morning were so packed with men, waggons, horses, bales, and lorries, that you could barely pick your way between them.

Since writing this an aeroplane has been circling over us with a loud buzz. The sergeant called up to me to put the lights out. We saw her light. There is much speculation as to who and what she was; she was not big enough for our big 'Bus', as she is called, who belongs to this place. No one seems ever to have seen one here at night before.

We are making flannel masks for the C.O. for our men.

Our fat little Gabrielle makes the most priceless soup out of the ration beef (which none of us are any good at) and carrots. She mothers us each individually, and cleans the house and keeps her wee kitchen spotless.

4 a.m. The 9.2's are just beginning to talk.

Here is a true story. One of our trenches at Givenchy was being pounded by German shells at the time of N. Ch. A man saw his brother killed on one side of him and another man on the other. He went on shooting over the parapet; then the parapet got knocked about, and still he wasn't hit. He seized his brother's body and the other man's and built them up into the parapet with sandbags, and went on shooting.

When the stress was over and he could leave off, he looked round and saw what he was leaning against. 'Who did that?' he said. And they told him.

They get awfully sick at the big-print headlines in some of the papers – 'The Hill 60 Thrill'!

'Thrill, indeed! There's nothing thrilling about ploughing over parapets into a machine-gun, with high explosives bursting round you, – it's merely beastly,' said a boy this evening, who is all over shrapnel splinters.

Saturday, May 8th, 9 a.m.

This is Der Tag. Could anybody go to bed and undress?

I have been cutting dressings all night. One of the most stabbing things in this war is seeing the lines of empty motor ambulances going up to bring down the wrecks who at this moment are sound and fit, and all absolutely ready to be turned into wrecks.

10.30 p.m. Der Tag was a wash-out, but it is to begin at 1.15 to-night. (It didn't!)

The tension is more up than ever. A boy who has just come in with a poisoned heel (broken-hearted because he is out of it, while his battalion moves up) says, 'You'll be having them in in cartloads over this.'

Sunday, May 9th, 1.30 a.m.

The Lions are roaring in full blast and lighting up the sky.

Have been busy to-night with an operation case who is needing a lot of special nursing, and some admissions – one in at 11 p.m., who was only wounded at 9 o'clock. I hope these magnificent roars and rumblings are making a mess of the barbed wire and German trenches. There seems to be a pretty general opinion that they will retaliate by dropping them into this place if they have time, and pulverising it like Ypres.

5.25 a.m. It has begun. It is awful – continuous and earthquaking.

9.30 a.m. – In bed. The last ten minutes of 'Rapid' did its damnedest and then began again, and we are still thundering hell into the German lines.

It began before 5 with a fearful pounding from the French on our right, and hasn't left off since.

Had a busy night with my operation case and the others (he is doing fine), and in every spare second getting ready for the rush. The M.O.'s were astir very early; the A.D.M.S. came to count empty beds. It is to-night they'll be coming in.

Must try and sleep. But who could yesterday and to-day?

Monday, May 10th, 9.30 a.m.

We have had a night of it. Every Field Ambulance, barge,

Clearing Hospital, and train are blocked with them. The M.O.'s neither eat nor sleep. I got up early yesterday and went down to the barge to see if they wanted any extra help (as the other two were coping with the wounded officers), and had a grim afternoon and evening there. One M.O., no Sisters, four trained orderlies, and some other men were there. It was packed with all the worst cases – dying and bleeding and groaning. After five hours we had three-fourths of them out of their blood-soaked clothes, dressed, fed, hæmorrhage stopped, hands and faces washed, and some asleep. Two died, and more were dying. They all worked like bricks. The M.O., and another from the other barge which hadn't filled up, sent up to the O.D.S., when my hour for night duty there came, to ask if I could stay, and got leave. At 11 p.m. four Sisters arrived (I don't know how – they'd been wired for), two for each barge; so I handed over to them and went to the O.D.S. to relieve the other two there for night duty. The place was unrecognisable: every corner of

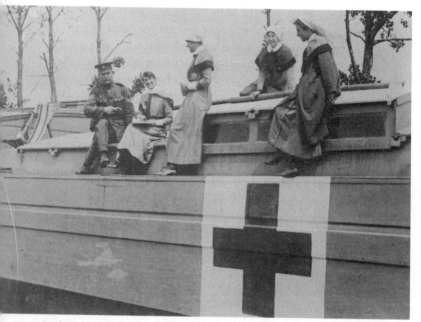

Red Cross nurses on a hospital barge.

every floor filled with wounded officers – some sitting up and some all over wounds, and three dying and others critical; and they still kept coming in. They were all awfully good strewing about the floor – some soaked to the skin from wet shell holes – on their stretchers, waiting to be put to bed.

One had had 'such a jolly Sunday afternoon' lying in a shell hole with six inches of water in it and a dead man, digging himself in deeper with his trench tool whenever the shells burst near him. He was hit in the stomach.

One officer saw the enemy through a periscope sniping at our wounded.

4 p.m. In bed. It seems quiet to-day; there are so few guns to be heard, and not so many ambulances coming. All except the hopeless cases will have been evacuated by now from all the Field Hospitals. There was a block last night, and none could be sent on. The Clearing Hospitals were full, and no trains in.

Those four Sisters from the base had a weird arrival at the barge last night in a car at 11 p.m. It was a black dark night, big guns going, and a sudden descent down a ladder into that Nelson's cockpit. They were awfully bucked when we said, 'Oh, I am glad you have come.' They buckled to and set to work right off. The cook, who had been helping magnificently in the ward, was running after me with hot cocoa (breakfast was my last meal, except a cup of tea), and promised to give them some. One wounded of the Munsters there said he didn't mind nothink now – he'd seen so many dead Germans as he never thought on. As always, they have lost thousands, but they come on like ants.

They have only had about seven new cases to-day at the O.D.S., but two of last night's have died. A Padre was with them.

They had no market this morning, for fear of bombs from aeroplanes. There's been no shelling into the town.

Tuesday, May 11th, 6.30 p.m.
In bed. I went to bed pretty tired this morning after an awful night (only a few of the less seriously wounded had

been evacuated yesterday, and all the worst ones, of course, left), and slept like a top from 10.30 to 5, and feel as fit as anything after it.

The fighting seems to have stopped now, and no more have come in to-day. Last night a stiff muddy figure, all bandages and straw, on the stretcher was brought in. I asked the boy how many wounds? 'Oh, only five,' he said cheerfully. 'Nice clean wounds – machine-gun – all in and out again!'

The Padre came at 7.30 and had a Celebration in each ward, but I was too busy to take any notice of it.

One of these officers was hit by a German shell on Sunday morning early, soon after our bombardment began. He crawled about till he was hit again twice by other shells, and then lay there all that day and all that night, with one drink from another wounded's water-bottle; every one else was either dead or wounded round him. Next morning his servant found him and got stretcher-bearers, and he got here.

I don't know how they live through that.

Wednesday, May 12th, 6.30 p.m.
Slept very well. I hear from Gabrielle that they have had a hard day at the O.D.S.; no new cases, but all the bad ones very ill.

My little room is crammed with enormous lilac, white and purple, from our wee garden, which I am going to take to our graves to-morrow in jam tins.

Thursday, May 13th, 11 a.m.
Can't face the graves to-day; have had an awful night; three died during the night. I found the boy who brought his officer in from between the German line and ours, on Sunday night, crying this morning over the still figure under a brown blanket on a stretcher.

Of the other two, brought straight in from the other dressing station, one only lived long enough to be put to bed, and the other died on his stretcher in the hall.

The O.C. said last night, 'Now this War has come we've got to tackle it with our gloves off,' but it takes some tackling. It seems so much nearer, and more murderous somehow in this Field Ambulance atmosphere even than it did on the train with all the successive hundreds.

We can see Notre Dame de Lorette from here; the Chapel and Fort stand high up in that flat maze of slag-heaps, mine-heads, and sugar-factories just behind the line on the right.

9 p.m., O.D.S. Everything very quiet here.

A gunner just admitted says there will probably be another big bombardment to-morrow morning, and after that another attack, and after that I suppose some more for us.

Another says that the charge of the Black Watch on Sunday was a marvellous thing. They went into it playing the pipes! The Major who led it handed somebody his stick, as he 'probably shouldn't want it again.'

It is very wet to-night, but they go up to the trenches singing Ragtime, some song about 'We are always – respected – wherever we go'. And another about 'Sing a song – a song with me. Come along – along with me'.

11 p.m. Just heard a shell burst, first the whistling scream, and then the bang – wonder where? There was another about an hour ago, but I didn't hear the whistle of that – only the bang. I shouldn't have known what the whistle was if I hadn't heard it at Braisne. It goes in a curve. All the men on the top floor have been sent down to sleep in the cellar; another shell has busted.

12.15. Just had another, right overhead; all the patients are asleep, luckily.

1.30 p.m. There was one more, near enough to make you jump, and a few more too far off to hear the whistling. A sleepy major has just waked up and said, 'Did you hear the shells? Blackguards, aren't they?'

The sky on the battle line to-night is the weirdest sight; our guns are very busy, and they are making yellow flashes like huge sheets of summer lightning. Then the star-shells rise, burst, and light up a large area, while a big searchlight plays slowly on the clouds. It is all very beautiful when you don't think what it means.

Two more – the last very loud and close. It is somehow much more alarming than Braisne, perhaps because it is among buildings, and because one knows so much more what they mean.

Another – the other side of the building.

An ambulance has been called out, so some one must have been hit; I've lost count of how many they've dropped, but they could hardly fail to do some damage.

5 a.m. Daylight – soaking wet, and no more shells since 2 a.m. We have admitted seven officers to-night; the last – just in – says there have been five people wounded in the town by this peppering – one killed. I don't know if civilians or soldiers.

That bombardment on Sunday morning was the biggest any one has ever heard – more guns on smaller space, and more shells per minute.

Nine officers have 'died of wounds' here since Sunday, and the tenth will not live to see daylight. There is an attack on to-night. This has been a ghastly week, and now it is beginning again.

The other two Sisters had quite a nasty time last night lying in bed, waiting for the shells to burst in their rooms. They do sound exactly as if they are coming your way and nowhere else!

I rather think they are dropping some in again to-night, but they are not close enough to hear the whistle, only the bangs.

There is an officer in to-night with a wound in the hand and shoulder from a shell which killed eleven of his men, and another who went to see four of his platoon in a house at the exact moment when a percussion shell went on the same errand; the whole house sat down, and the five were wounded – none killed.

Saturday, May 15th, 10 p.m.

Tension up again like last Saturday. Another TAG is happening to-morrow. Everyone except three sick downstairs has been evacuated, and they have made accommodation for 1000 at the French Hospital, which is the 4th F.A. main dressing station, and headquarters. All officers, whether seriously or slightly wounded, are to be taken there to be dressed by the M.O.'s in the specially-arranged dressing-rooms, and then sent on to us to be put to bed and coped with.

Now we have got some French batteries of 75's in our lines to pound the earthworks which protect the enemy's buried machine-guns, which are the most murderous and deadly of all their clever arrangements, and to stop up the holes through which they are fired. We have also got more Divisions in it along the same front, and our heavy guns and all our batteries in better positions.

Some more regiments have been called up in a hurry, and empty ammunition-carts are galloping back already.

This morning I took some white lilac to the graves of our 12 officers who 'died of wounds'. Their names and regiments were on their crosses, and 'Died of wounds.—F.A.', and R.I.P. It was better to see them like that Pro Patria than in those few awful days here.

10.30. Just admitted a gunner suffering from shock alone – no wound – completely knocked out; he can't tell you his name, or stand, or even sit up, but just shivers and shudders. Now he is warm in bed, he can say 'Thank you'. I wonder what exactly did it.

The arrangements the — F.A. happen to have the use of at the French Hospital, with its up-to-date modern operating theatre for tackling the wounds in a strictly aseptic and scientific way within a few hours of the men being hit, are a tremendous help.

Certainly the ones who pass through No.— get a better chance of early recovery without long complications than most of those we got on the train. And while they are awaiting evacuation to the Clearing Hospitals they have every chance, both here and at the French Hospital, where all the trained orderlies except two are on duty, and practically all the M.O.'s. But, of course, there are a great many of the seriously wounded that no amount of aseptic and skilled surgery or nursing can save.

Sunday, 11.30 a.m.*May 16th.*
They began coming in at 3.30, and by 8 a.m. the place was full to bursting. We managed to get all the stretcher cases to bed, and as many of the others as we had beds for, without sending for the other two Sisters, who came on at 8.15, and are now coping. Most of them were very cheery, because things seem to

be going well. Two lines of trenches taken, all the wire cut, and some of the earthworks down; but it is always an expensive business even when successful – only then nobody minds the expense. There are hundreds more to come in, and the seriously wounded generally get brought in last, because they can't get up and run, but have to hide in trenches and shell holes. One man, wounded on Sunday and found on Friday night, had kept himself alive on dead men's emergency rations. They were all sopping wet with blood or mud or both.

The —— lost heavily. I heard one officer say, 'They drove us back five times.'

After breakfast I went to the Cathedral, and then boldly bearded the big dressing station at the French Hospital, where all the dressings are done and the men evacuated, armed with a huge linen bag of cigarettes, chocolate, and writing-cases which came last night. I met the C.O., who said I could have a look round, and then rowed me for not being in bed, and said we should be busy to-night and for some time. It was very interesting, and if you brought your reason to bear on it, not too horrible.

Every corridor, waiting-room, ward, and passage was filled with them, the stretchers waiting their turn on the floors, and the walking cases (which on the A.T. we used to call the sitting-ups) in groups and queues. No one was fussing, but all were working at full pitch; and very few of the men were groaning, but nearly all were gruesomely covered with blood. And they look pretty awful on the bare gory stretchers, with no pillows or blankets, just as they are picked up on the field. Many are asleep from exhaustion.

What cheered me was one ward full of last Sunday's bad cases, all in bed, and very cheery and doing well. They loved the writing-cases, &c., and said it was like Xmas, and they wouldn't want to leave 'ere now.

A great many of this morning's had already been evacuated, and they were still pouring in. One has to remember that a great many get quite well, though many have a ghastly time in store for them in hospital.

The barge is in the canal again taking in the non-jolters.

Some stalwart young Tommies at No. 4 were talking about the prisoners. They told me there weren't many taken, because they found one in a Jock's uniform.

I've drawn my curtain so that I can't see those hateful motor ambulances coming in slowly full, and going back empty fast, and must go to sleep. I simply loathe the sight of those M.A.'s, admirable inventions though they are. Had a look into a lovely lorry full of 100-lb. shells in the square.

7 p.m. Only one officer has died at the O.D.S. to-day, but there are two or three who will die. They have evacuated, and filled up three times already.

The news from the 'scene of operations' is still good, so they are all still cheerful. The difference to the wounded that makes is extraordinary. That is why last Sunday's show was such a black blight to them and to us.

Monday, May 17th, 10 a.m.
Another night of horrors; one more died, and two young boys came in who will die; one is a Gordon Highlander of 18, who says 'that's glorious' when you put him to bed.

It was a long whirl of stretchers, and pitiful heaps on them. The sergeant stayed up helping till 3, and a boy from the kitchen stayed up all night on his own, helping.

In the middle of the worst rush the sergeant said to me, 'You know they're shelling the town again?' and at that minute swoop bang came a big one; and we looked at each other over the stretcher with the same picture in our mind's eyes of shells dropping in amongst the wounded, who are all over the town. I hadn't heard them – too busy – but they didn't go on long.

The Boches have been heavily shelling our trenches all day.

One boy said suddenly, when I was attending to his leg, 'Aren't you very foolish to be staying up here?' 'Oh, sorry,' he said; 'I was dreaming you were in the front line of trenches bandaging people up!'

Our big guns have been making the building shake all night. The Germans are trying to get their trenches back by counter-attacking.

Tuesday, May 18th, is it? 1 a.m., *in bed.*

It has been about the worst night of all the worst nights. I found the wards packed with bad cases, the boy of 18 dead, and the other boy died half an hour after I came on. Two more died during the night, two lots were evacuated, and had to be dug out of their fixings-up in bed and settled on stretchers, and all night they brought fresh ones in, drenched and soaked with clayey mud in spadefuls, and clammy with cold.

Wednesday, May 19th, 12 noon.

Mr —— has been working at No.— at full pitch for twenty-four hours on end, and had just got into bed when they sent for him there again. They are all nearly dead, and so are the orderlies at both places; but they never dream of grousing or shirking, as they know there's not another man to be had.

Two more officers died last night, and three more were dying.

The Padre came and had a Celebration in my ward. Three R.A.M.C. officers are in badly wounded. They are extraordinarily good.

Friday, 21st May, 3 a.m.

Last night the rush began to abate; no one died, and only one came in – a general smash-up; he died to-night, and a very dear boy died to-day. I've lost count now of how many have died – I think about twenty-four.

The Guards' Brigade here went by to-night from the trenches to rest, singing 'Here we are again', and the song about 'The girls declare I am a funny man!'

11 a.m. The little Canadian Sister has just been recalled, I'm sorry to say, but probably we shall get another one. Five Canadian officers came in last night. The guns are making the dickens of a noise, very loud and sudden. Yesterday they shelled the town again, and two more *soldats anglais* were wounded.

Saturday, May 22nd, 6.30 a.m.

Things have been happening at a great pace since the above, and we are now in our camp-beds in an empty attic at the top of an old château about three miles back, which is No.— C.H., at ——.

Just as I was thinking of getting up yesterday evening they began putting shells over into the town, and soon they were raining in three at a time. My little room here is a sort of lean-to over the kitchen with no room above it; so I cleared out to dress in one of the others, and didn't stop to wash. Gabrielle came running up to fetch me downstairs. At the hospital, which was only about 200 yards down the road, the wounded officers were thinking it was about time Capt. —— moved his Field Ambulance. One boy by the window had got some *débris* in his eye from the nearest shell, which burst in my blackbird's garden, or rather on the doorstep opposite. (That was the one that got me out of bed rather rapidly.) The orders soon came to evacuate all the patients. At the French Hospital, about six minutes away, three wounded had been hit in a M.A. coming in, and the Officers' Mess had one (none of them were in), and they were dropping all round it. Then the order came from the D.D.M.S. to the A.D.M.S. to evacuate the whole of the —th, —th, and —th Field Ambulances, and within about two hours this was done.

Everybody got the patients ready, fixed up their dressings and splints, gave them all morphia, and got them on to their stretchers.

The evacuation was jolly well done; their servants appeared by magic, each with every spot of kit and belongings his officer came in with (they are in *all* cases checked by the Sergeant on admission, no matter what the rush is), and the place was empty in an hour. The din of our guns, which were bombarding heavily, and the German guns, which are bombarding us at a great pace, and the whistle and bang of the shells that came over while this was going on, was a din to remember.

Then we went back to our billet to hurl our belongings into our baggage, and came away with the A.D.M.S. and his Staff-

Major in their two touring-cars. The Division is back resting somewhere near here. We got to bed about 2 a.m. after tea and bread and butter downstairs, but slept very little owing to the noise of the guns, which shake and rattle the windows every minute.

We don't know what happens next.

At about four this morning I heard a nightingale trilling in the garden.

2 p.m. In the Château garden. It is a glorious spot, with kitchen garden, park, moat bridge, and a huge wilderness up-and-down plantation round it, full of lilac, copper beeches, and flowering trees I've never seen before, and birds and butterflies and buttercups. You look across and see the red-brick Château surrounded by thick lines of tents, and hear the everlasting incessant thudding and banging of the guns, and realise that it is not a French country house but a Casualty Clearing Hospital, with empty – once polished – floors filled with stretchers, where the worst cases still are, and some left empty for the incoming convoys. Over two thousand have passed through since Sunday week. The contrast between the shady garden where I'm lazing now on rugs and cushions, with innumerable birds, including a nightingale, singing and nesting, and the nerve-racking sound of the guns and the look of the place inside, is overwhelming. It is in three Divisions – the house for the worst cases – and there are tent Sections and the straw-sheds and two schools in the village. We had our lunch at a sort of inn in the village. I've never hated the sound of the guns so much; they are almost unbearable.

It is a good thing for us to have this sudden rest. I don't know for how long or what happens next.

The General of the Division had a narrow escape after we left last night. The roof of his house was blown off, just at the time he would have been there, only he was a little late, but an officer was killed; six shells came into the garden, and the seventh burst at his feet and killed him as he was standing at the door. I'm glad they got the wounded away in time. Aeroplanes are buzzing overhead. The Aerodrome is here,

French monoplanes chiefly as far as one can see.

10 p.m., *in bed*. We have now been temporarily attached to the Staff here.

Miss —— has given me charge of the Tent Section, which can take eighty lying down.

Whitsunday, 1915.

In bed – in my tent, not a bell, but an Indian tent big enough for two comfortably. I share with S——. We have nothing but the camp furniture we took out, but will acquire a few Red Cross boxes as cupboards to-morrow. It is a peerless night with a young moon and a soft wind, frogs croaking, guns banging, and a nightingale trilling.

It has been a funny day, dazzling sun, very few patients.

Whit-Monday.

Very few in to-day again. I have only six, and am making the most of the chance of a rest in the garden; one doesn't realise till after a rush how useful a rest can be. There has been a fearful bombardment going on all last night and yesterday and to-day; it is a continual roar, and in the night is maddening to listen to; you can't forget the war. Mosquitoes, nightingales, frogs, and two horses also helped to make the night interesting.

8.30 p.m. Waiting for supper. Wounded have been coming in, and we've had a busy afternoon and evening.

Wednesday, May 26th.

No time to write yesterday; had a typical Clearing Hospital Field Day. The left-out-in-the-field wounded (mostly Canadians) had at last been picked up and came pouring in. I had my Tent Section of eighty beds nearly full, and we coped in a broiling sun till we sweltered into little spots of grease, finishing up with five operations in the little operating tent.

The poor exhausted Canadians were extraordinarily brave and uncomplaining. They are evacuated the same day or the next morning, such as can be got away to survive the journey, but some of the worst have to stay.

In the middle of it all at 5 p.m. orders came for me to join No.— Ambulance Train for duty, but I didn't leave till this morning at nine, and am now on No.— A.T. on way down to old Boulogne again.

Later. These orders were afterwards cancelled, and I am for duty at a Base Hospital.

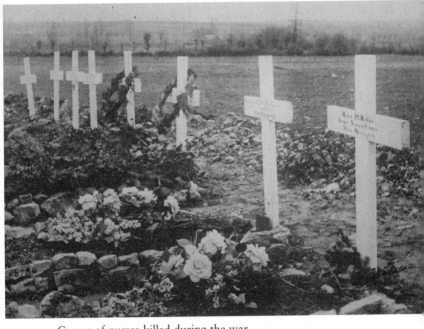

Graves of nurses killed during the war.

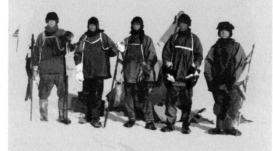

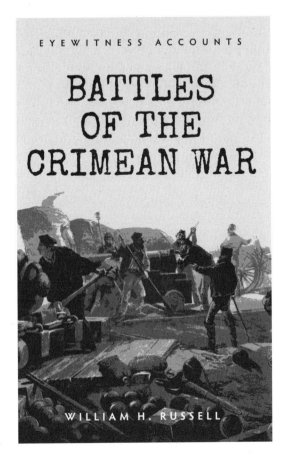

Battles of the Crimean War
William H. Russell

This book reprints Russell's vivid accounts of the battlefields of the
Alma, Sevastapol, Balaclava and Inkerman.

978 1 4456 3789 1
224 pages, illustrated

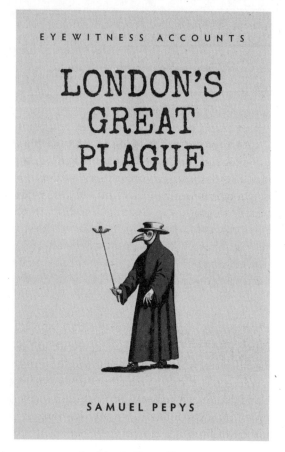